SOAP MAKING

Recipies, Techniques, Step by Step
Instruction to Create Natural Homemade
Soap Using Essential Oils, Herbs
and Spices

By
Ella Diamond

Table of Contents

Chapter One: Soap Background 1

    The Kettle Process 4

Introduction 8

    Safety equipment 9

    Weighing scale...9

    Quart Heat-Safe Containers 9

    Stainless steel pot...10

    3-quart stainless steel sauce pan................................10

    Wooden or silicone utensils......................................10

    Thermometers...10

    Molds 10

    Wax paper...11

    Tape 11

    Soap cutter or knife...11

    Soap Making and Its Advantages in Our Lives 15

Chapter Two : 18Soap Making Safety 18

    How to Make Handmade Soap Safely...................................19

    Understanding The Ingredients.............................20

    Using Accurate Measurements 22

    Keeping Your Eyes Safe 24

    Keeping Your Skin Safe 25

    Breathing Clean Air...26

    Having Emergency Backup On Hand....................28

    Creating A Plan & Following A Process..................29

Chapter Three : Choose the right soapmaking equipment 33

    Accurate scale...38

    Safety goggles and rubber gloves..............................39

Chapter Four : The Importance Things To know About
Soap Making 42

Chapter Five : How to Blend Essential Oils For Natural Beauty and Soap Making 45

Tips to Using Essential and Fragile Oils When Making Soap 47

Use cold process soap making. 47

Do not add the essential oils too early 48

Mix fragile oils with carrier oils. 48

Scenting Your 49

Beginners Guide To Soap Making 51

Chapter Six : How To Make Liquid Soap 54

Melt And Pour Process 56

Melt And Pour Soap Making Equipment And Ingredients 59

Essential Oils For Aromatherapy in Handmade Bath Products 62

Herbal Soap Making 66

How to Make Natural Soap 74

Homemade Soap Making Equipment 76

How to Make Soap for Hand & Body 78

Chapter Seven : Soap Making Recipe For the Holidays 86

Reasons to Make Handmade Soap 89

Types of Soap Making Molds You Can Work With 91

Soap Making Mold - Let Your Imagination Run Wild! 94

Organic Soap Making Supplies and Materials 96

Synthetic Soap - Coloring Option 99

Liquid Soap 102

Aromatherapy Soaps 104

Common Mistakes in the Soap Making Process 106

Making Heavenly Vanilla Soap Using The Melt and Pour Process 109

The Role of Glycerine in the Production of Soap 113

iii

The Benefits of Organic Soaps Without Toxicity 116

Hand Made Soaps - Advantages and Materials 118

The Truth Surrounding Homemade Soap Recipes Finally
Revealed 120

Starting a Soap Making Business at Home 123

Learning the Good Stuff About Soap Making 129

Chapter Eight : Best Homemade Soap Recipes: 132

Handmade Soap Recipes 135

Disclaimer 148

CHAPTER ONE

SOAP BACKGROUND

Soap is a combination of animal fat or plant oil and caustic soda. When dissolved in water, it breaks dirt away from surfaces. Through the ages soap has been used to cleanse, to cure skin sores, to dye hair, and as a salve or skin ointment. But today we generally use soap as a cleanser or perfume.

The exact origins of soap are unknown, though Roman sources claim it dates back to at least 600 B.C. , when Phoenicians prepared it from goat's tallow and wood ash. Soap was also made by the Celts, ancient inhabitants of Britain. Soap was used widely throughout the Roman empire, primarily as a medicine. Mention of soap as a cleanser does not appear until the second century A.D. By the eighth century, soap was common in France, Italy, and Spain, but it was rarely used in the rest of Europe until as late as the 17th century.

Manufacture of soap began in England around the end of the 12th century. Soap-makers had to pay a heavy tax on all the soap they produced. The tax collector locked the lids on soap boiling pans every night to prevent illegal soap manufacture after hours. Because of the high tax, soap was a luxury item, and it did not come into common use in England until after the tax was repealed in 1853. In the 19th century, soap was affordable and popular throughout Europe.

Early soap manufacturers simply boiled a solution of wood ash and animal fat. A foam substance formed at the top of the pot. When cooled, it hardened into soap. Around 1790, French soapmaker Nicolas Leblanc developed a method of extracting caustic soda (sodium hydroxide) from common table salt (sodium chloride), replacing the wood ash element of soap. The French chemist Eugene-Michel Chevreul put the soap-forming process (called in English saponification) into concrete chemical terms in 1823. In saponification, the animal fat, which is chemically neutral, splits into fatty acids, which react with alkali carbonates to form soap, leaving glycerin as a byproduct. Soap was made with industrial processes by the end of the 19th century, though people in rural areas, such as the pioneers in the western United States, continued to make soap at home.

Raw Materials

Soap requires two major raw materials: fat and alkali. The alkali most commonly used today is sodium hydroxide. Potassium hydroxide can also be used. Potassium-based soap creates a more water-soluble product than sodium-based soap, and so it is called "soft soap." Soft soap, alone or in combination with sodium-based soap, is commonly used in shaving products.

Animal fat in the past was obtained directly from a slaughterhouse. Modern soapmakers use fat that has been processed into fatty acids. This eliminates many impurities, and it produces as a byproduct water instead of glycerin. Many vegetable fats, including olive oil, palm kernel oil, and coconut oil, are also used in soap making.

Additives are used to enhance the color, texture, and scent of soap. Fragrances and perfumes are added to the soap mixture to cover the odor of dirt and to leave behind a fresh-smelling scent. Abrasives to enhance the texture of soap include talc, silica, and marble pumice (volcanic ash). Soap made without dye is a dull grey or brown color, but modern manufacturers color soap to make it more enticing to the consumer.

The Manufacturing

Process

The kettle method of making soap is still used today by small soap manufacturing companies. This process takes from four to eleven days to complete, and the quality of each batch is inconsistent due to the variety of oils used. Around 1940, engineers and scientists developed a more efficient manufacturing process, called the continuous process. This procedure is employed by large soap manufacturing companies all around the world today. Exactly as the name states, in the continuous process soap is produced continuously, rather than one batch at a time. Technicians have more control of the production in the continuous process, and the steps are much quicker than in the kettle method—it takes only about six hours to complete a batch of soap.

The Kettle Process

Boiling

Fats and alkali are melted in a kettle, which is a steel tank that can stand three stories high and hold several thousand pounds of material. Steam coils within the kettle heat the batch and bring it to a boil. After boiling, the mass thickens as the fat reacts with the alkali, producing soap and glycerin.

Salting

The soap and glycerin must now be separated. The mixture is treated with salt, causing the soap to rise to the top and the glycerin to settle to the bottom. The glycerin is extracted from the bottom of the kettle.

Strong change

To remove the small amounts of fat that have not saponified, a strong caustic solution is added to the kettle. This step in the process is called "strong change." The mass is brought to a boil again, and the last of the fat turns to soap. The batch may be given another salt treatment at this time, or the manufacturer may proceed to the next step.

Pitching

The next step is called "pitching." The soap in the kettle is boiled again with added water. The mass eventually separates into two layers. The top layer is called "neat soap," which is about 70% soap and 30% water. The lower layer, called "nigre," contains most of the impurities in the soap such as dirt and salt, as well as most of the water. The neat soap is taken off the top. The soap is then cooled. The finishing process is the Developed around 1940 and used by today's major soap-making companies, the above illustrations show the continuous process of making soap.

Developed around 1940 and used by today's major soap-making companies, the above illustrations show the continuous process of making soap. same as for soap made by the continuous process

The Continuous Process

Splitting

The first step of the continuous process splits natural fat into fatty acids and glycerin. The equipment used is a vertical stainless steel column with the diameter of a barrel called a hydrolizer. It may be as tall as 80 feet

(24 m). Pumps and meters attached to the column allow precise measurements and control of the process. Molten fat is pumped into one end of the column, while at the other end water at high temperature (266°F [130°C]) and pressure is introduced. This splits the fat into its two components. The fatty acid and glycerin are pumped out continuously as more fat and water enter. The fatty acids are then distilled for purification.

Mixing

The purified fatty acids are next mixed with a precise amount of alkali to form soap. Other ingredients such as abrasives and fragrance are also mixed in. The hot liquid soap may be then whipped to incorporate air.

Cooling and finishing

The soap may be poured into molds and allowed to harden into a large slab. It may also be cooled in a special freezer. The slab is cut into smaller pieces of bar size, which are then stamped and wrapped. The entire continuous process, from splitting to finishing, can be accomplished in several hours.

Milling

Most toiletry soap undergoes additional processing called milling. The milled bar lathers up better and has a finer consistency than non-milled soap. The cooled soap is fed through several sets of heavy rollers (mills), which crush and knead it. Perfumes can best be incorporated at this time because their volatile oils do not evaporate in the cold mixture. After the soap emerges from the mills, it is pressed into a smooth cylinder and extruded. The extruded soap is cut into bar size, stamped and wrapped.

By products

Glycerin is a very useful byproduct of soap manufacture. It is used to make hand lotion, drugs, and nitroglycerin, the main component of explosives such as dynamite.

INTRODUCTION

The Soap making hobby and business has soared rapidly for the past years which brought about the growth of soap making classes. What is good about attending school is that they are not teaching only how to make soap bars but also liquid soaps. A soap making class is considered efficient, if safety equipment, molds and recipes are included in the module.

If your goal in learning how to make soap is to create a profitable business out of it take some time also to include a business class while you are there. Business is not just merely selling, you have to be equipped with sufficient knowledge about marketing, inventory, product selection, pricing and the like. Making soap nowadays is very competitive and one must know how to stand out from the rest.

There is so much to learn when it comes to starting a business making and selling soap. Taking it one step at a time will ensure success. Learn the skill of making soap first and then start the business side to make money from your talents.

Soap making is one of the most sought for pleasurable past time by many especially to housewives. Surprisingly, this hobby does not end there, many young people are also doing it. Nowadays, people are more drawn to use natural soap which opened a lot of doors to homemade soap enthusiast.

Making soap is fun and challenging and the soap making supply needed is just right in front of you. Look around your house and you will find the basic tools you need. Perhaps there are a few that may not be in your house but are easy to obtain in craft stores.

What are the most important and basic equipment that a novice must have?

Safety equipment

This is a must have to all 'soap enthusiasts'. Always wear rubber gloves and goggles when making soap to protect skin and eyes from lye solution and even caustic raw material of soap. Safety equipment is readily available in any hardware or supermarkets.

Weighing scale

It is best if the measuring scale can measure in two ways, grams and ounces. If this is not possible then the use of two kinds of scales is best.

Quart Heat-Safe Containers

Containers used in soap making must be heat-resistant. Some plastics may react to the heat and may cause chemical reaction.

Stainless steel pot

This is used in melting soap and blending other ingredients such as lye, oils, additives, and fats. Use large pots to be able to accommodate all mixtures.

3-quart stainless steel sauce pan

Saucepans are one of the soap making supplies that are used to melt solid oils, fats and additives.

Wooden or silicone utensils

Both are suitable in soap making however there is one drawback when using wood. Wooden utensils tend to corrode and chip off when constantly exposed to soap solutions. So if soap making is done on a regular basis, it is better to use silicone utensils.

Thermometers

Use two accurate thermometers, one for measuring lye and one for measuring oils.

Molds

Molds can be in different shapes. You can use individually molds or wooden molds in bars. A soap maker can also become creative in this aspect of soap making by looking for old things in your garage that can be used as molds. It is inexpensive yet unique.

Wax paper

This can be used as a layering inside the mold for ease of taking the soap out of the mold. This can also be used to cover the top of the mold while waiting for its curing time to prevent heat from releasing abruptly. Wax papers can be easily bought in supermarkets.

Tape

Masking tapes are used to keep wax paper in place on the mold.

Soap cutter or knife

Soap cutters are used for cutting big rectangular bars of soap, though a knife may be used if the soaps are only for family use. Soap cutters are preferable when it is to be sold.

This is the basic soap making supply an soap enthusiast must have before starting his or her endeavor. As mentioned it is not hard or expensive since this tools are readily available at home.

Soap like food and clothes is one of the essentials of life and making soap is a good skill to learn especially soap making at home because it not only means you have the exact mixture and texture you want but also it means saving money.

Soap comes in different shapes, sizes, texture and color, and even now there also all types of liquid soaps around to choose from.

However, the mean bone of contention is that most of the soap available in the market don't meet the exact requirements of the users i.e. they might meet all our requirements but be lacking in one specific area e.g. might be too hard or too soft, might not meet our fantasy in terms of shape, etc.

The question therefore is why do you have to compromise having your favorite fragrance simply because it does not come in the pink or blue color you would have preferred or settle down for a hard soap simple because that is the only available that includes the soothing oils you so much desire or that was medically recommended for you.

So if you don't feel like compromising what do you do? Make your own soap? But surely that would be difficult! Very expensive! Really, really time consuming! The idea of making soap at home raises so many questions in our minds.

However, the good news is that all the above issues are myths and much more that your minds could think of. Making soap at home is very easy, cheap, can be done around your other activities at home and above all provides you with all the different specific choices you require in your soap.

The recipe for soap making is a derivative of either oils or fats. Most soap is based on sodium compounds derived from animal fats. A lot of soaps are also made using vegetable fats these could be as simply as olive oil. Most of the things needed for making soap is available at home and all that is needed is the know how which in itself is not something you need to get a college degree for but rather a little inexpensive book would do the trick.

The soap is a surfactant used in conjunction with water for washing and cleaning, which traditionally comes either in solid bars or in the form of a thick liquid. Soap consists of sodium or potassium salts of fatty acids and is gained by reacting common oils or fats with a strong alkaline solution in a process known as saponification. The fats are hydrolyzed by the base, docile alkali salts of fatty acids and glycerol. The most accepted soap making process today is the cold process method, where fats such as olive oil react with lye, whereas some soapers use the historical hot process.

To initiate soap making, you will feel like grating all your soap into the small specks. Then place all your flakes into the glass bowl that can be furthermore placed in the double boiler; and as double boiler heats up, all you will want is to combine your shredded soap piece. Put some vegetable oils and scents at this end, making it certain that all things are also integrated. Crack up the soap clomps that have figure and persist to heat pending the soap enter the string phase, and at this point in time, the soap will even solidify quickly. Remove the pot from the heat resource as it rapidly append in the fragrances, coloring, herbs, and elective items in meticulous order; and ladling into the molds also lets it to cure.

There is a lot of soap making procedures out there that can help you create soap. The first method for soap making is known as the cold process soap making where it requires materials such as the pot made from stainless steel that is large enough, the rubber gloves, the kitchen thermometers, the lye, scale, mold, the measuring cups, cardboard, coconut oil, olive oil, plastic bags, fragrances, and distilled water. The cold procedure is named from the common low level temperatures that are exploited to grind this sort of soap.

The art or hobby of making soap needs a soap maker to have the proper materials for their craft. Molds for soap making and other supplies can simply be found in different places, as long as you know what it is you're looking for. In fact, a lot of new soap makers uncover that they don't really need to purchase anything new in order to start their hobby. Making soap recipe with no usage of lye completely is not viable so it's completely your desire to use lye in your soap production process or you feel like trying your hands in glycerine based soaps.

By enclosing soap scraps, you can utilize this hand milled soap creation method, which is called the soap re-batching which you would like modifying into new tavern of the soap. For this, you will need a grater, the mold, soap scraps, dyes, fragrance, and other additives. The best kind of method for this type of soap making is the cold process.

Soap Making and Its Advantages in Our Lives

People have already made the wise decision of switching to organic beauty products. Chemicals used in these products may harm the skin when used. Particularly for soaps, we use them on a daily basis so we have to make sure that the product that we are using is safe on the skin.

The art of soap making is indeed an interesting activity that you should try out. This allows you to make organic soaps that are safe for the skin. You do not have to worry about your skin drying as well as getting allergies and rashes. All of the ingredients that you will use are practically natural so there is no need to worry about these anymore. Everything that you are looking for in a safe soap to use can be found in these kinds of soaps.

Soap is practically made through the process of

saponification. It is practically the hydrolysis of fatty acid esters with a base to form the carbolyxate soaps. In simple terms, you just have to mix animal or vegetable oil with lye to form your soaps. This is how simple soaps are made. You can definitely enjoy this activity as you make soaps that you can actually use.

Start soap making by the easiest method- the 'melt and pour' method. This type of soap making method is actually very simple to follow. All that you have to do is buy the soap base. It just has to be melted before you add any of the additives for the soap. Once it has created a homogenous mixture, you can now have the soap harden. As soon as it does, you can start using what you made.

The secret to having an effective soap is picking the right natural oils to use for it. Top choices for these are coconut oil, palm oil and olive oil. The advantage of using these in your soaps is that it cleanses the body without drying up.

You can rely on your creativity if you really want to make beautiful soaps. There are a lot of molds that you can use for soaps. These come in different shapes and sizes. You can take a visit to your favorite hobby store or even pick up a baking pan. You can even buy cookie cutters to cut out the soaps that you have made. It is all up to you on how you want to decorate your soaps.

Soap making is not just an activity that you can play with. Since you are handling dangerous raw materials, you have to make sure that you have protective covering. Never handle lye without the proper safety gear such as goggles, apron and even gas mask.

Organic handmade soaps are very fun to use! Especially if you made them from scratch, you will definitely enjoy using them. Switch to the safer alternative when using soaps. Do not let your skin get harmed. If you want beautiful skin, switch to only the natural choice.

CHAPTER TWO

SOAP MAKING SAFETY

Before even getting started making soap, ensure that you have all of your ingredients in your work area. Being prepared is one key factor in successful crafting. Once you get started, it is vital that you stay in your work area. Leaving certain ingredients such as lye out in the open can lead to very serious and dangerous situations. While you are prepping your area, it is also important to make sure that you have the proper soaping equipment, and it is in working order. Be sure to check the batteries on your scales to be certain they do not need changed before beginning the soap making process.

During the soap making process it is very important that you do not rush. Since soap making is a science, and you will want to ensure that everything is measured out exactly. Soap recipes are measured by weight units, not volume units. In other words, if a recipe calls for 8 oz. of coconut oil, you will need to weigh out 8 oz. of coconut oil on your scales. Take your time and move methodically. The best way to work is in an organized fashion. It is also very important that while you are making soap you are able to concentrate and work uninterrupted.

Soap-making can be a fun and rewarding hobby, its

also essential to have a good soap making guide as it can also be dangerous if the soap-maker doesn't research their materials, and take the proper precautions when making soap.

Lye is caustic and corrosive, meaning that it burns like acid when it comes into contact with skin or other surfaces.

Vinegar can help to neutralize lye when it is spilled, and prevent it from damaging surfaces, so it is a good idea to keep some on hand when working with lye.

Also, protect your work area with plastic bags, newspaper, or a vinyl tablecloth; make sure your work space is well-ventilated, because lye tends to evaporate quickly, and releases toxic fumes when it mixes with water. (If at all possible, it's best to make soap outside, so that spills and ventilation are non issues.)

Keep children and pets away from your work area and materials, and be sure to clean your equipment after each use; store lye properly in a tightly-sealed container, out of the reach of children and pets.

How to Make Handmade Soap Safely

While this should be a very basic topic for many soapmakers, I think that a lot of important parts of how to make handmade soap safely are typically overlooked. It took me years before I realized and put into place all the necessary safety measures I should have had from the start!

I hope this list of seven safety measures will help you get your wheels turning on how you can make cold process soap more safely!

Understanding The Ingredients

Throughout the hundreds of classes, talks, and workshops I've taught, tons of soapmakers have told me that their biggest obstacle in starting soapmaking was their fear of sodium hydroxide (lye). And while soapmakers always conquer that fear by diving in, they don't always do so armed with the proper information.

Consult a Safety Data Sheet for Each Ingredient You Use

To ensure you know how to safely use and store an ingredient, consult a SDS (Safety Data Sheet) for that ingredient from your supplier. If your supplier does not have a SDS for an ingredient available, you may want to ask them to supply you with one and consider finding a new supplier, if they will not give you one. In the mean time, you will likely be able to find and consult another supplier's SDS for the ingredient.

For instance, in the case of sodium hydroxide, many soapmakers for years have passed around the knowledge that they should clean lye solution spills and splashes with vinegar, when in reality, many SDS specifically state not to use any neutralizing agents! Here's two SDS examples for sodium hydroxide:

50% Sodium Hydroxide Solution (Lab Chem)

Sodium Hydroxide Beads (Sigma Aldrich)

You'll notice that if you spill lye solution on your skin, you should remove affected clothing, rinse with WATER, and consult a doctor or Poison Control. Splash it in your eye? Rinse with water. Get it in your mouth? Rinse with water. Only in the event of a small liquid spill does it ever recommend neutralizing (and even then, a spill kit is preferred), followed by rinsing with lots of water!

Research Your Ingredients Independently Before Using Them

Besides consulting a SDS before you use an ingredient, you should also do your research! Should you be using the ingredient in the manner that you plan? Is it safe to use the ingredient? With the ingredient react to another ingredient or react in the environment of the formulation? "I didn't know" isn't an appropriate response to improper ingredient usage! It's your job as a formulator to know.

Using Accurate Measurements

I'm often asked for the number of drops or how many cups of an ingredient to use in my tutorials, and the answer is always: I don't know, you should be weighing your ingredients! Measuring your ingredients by volume makes it extremely easy to use inaccurate amounts of an ingredient in a formula. You should always weigh your ingredients on an accurate digital scale for precision.

When manufacturing for resale, this includes your colorants and other additives! When I first started my business, I weighed everything to make the first batch of a product and entered those weights in my Soapmaker records. From there on out, all ingredients were weighed, even micas, natural colorants, etc. So, why do we use volume measurements for tutorials and as hobbyist? Most likely because it's easier and a lot of hobby soapmakers do not have a robust scale that can weigh small amounts of ingredients.

Keeping Your Scale Accurate

Once you have a quality digital scale to weigh your ingredients, it's not a set and forget it scenario! In order to make handmade soap safely time after time, your scale needs to remain accurate. How do you do that? Check it for accuracy often, and calibrate your scale periodically or as needed.

Most scales have a calibration mode, so if you wish to calibrate a scale yourself, refer to your scales manual. Note: it is direly important that you follow the directions exactly! You will need an accurate weight specifically for calibration. For instance, to calibrate a My Weigh KD-8000:

You need a 5 kg calibration weight

Turn the scale off and place it on a stable flat surface.

Press and hold the Power button and the MODE button at the same time, release both keys, and wait for the display to show CALE.

Place the 5 kg weight on the scale, wait three seconds, and press TARE. Wait for the display to read PASS, and then remove the 5 kg weight.

You'll notice that a calibration weight costs as much or more than the cost of this particular scale, especially depending on the class of the calibration weight!

If you are a hobbyist, you may purchase a smaller lower class calibration weight and check your scale for relative accuracy periodically. If your scale weighs a calibration weight inaccurately, you know it's time to either calibrate your scale or purchase a new one. For instance, a KD-8000 should remain accurate throughout it's lifetime (according to the manufacturer), and is calibrated during the manufacturing process, however, it's important to follow up and check it yourself.

Do you need your scale inspected?

If you are in business, you may need to register or obtain a license for your scale or have it inspected by your state's Department of Weights and Measures. For instance, in Arizona, a license is required for any commercial weighing, measuring or counting device used for commercial purposes in this state. And every scale used for commercial purposes requires having a NTEP Certificate of Conformance.

Keep Yourself in Check

To create a system of checks and balances, I highly recommend weighing each container you use in soapmaking and keeping a list handy. If you forget to tare your scale, it's as easy as checking your list and subtracting the weight of the container. Knowing the weight of your molds also makes it possible to weigh a finished batch, and determine if you are missing an oil.

Keeping Your Eyes Safe

Most soapmakers have seen the reasons for this safety measure first hand, with a splash of lye solution, a splatter of raw soap, or the sheer amount of particles that fly into the air while using colorants or making lye solution. So, it's safe to say that most soapmakers know they need to protect their peepers – yay!

Both lye solution and raw soap are caustic in nature and can severely injure a soapmaker. It goes without saying that wearing safety glasses or goggles will help prevent any eye injuries. Unless you are some kind of weird regenerating scientific anomaly, you shouldn't be throwing caution to the wind when it comes to protecting them.

From the most basic safety glasses to my favorite, onion goggles, to more heavy duty protection in face shields or full safety goggles, there is an endless array of options to protect your eyes.

Technically, you should be using coverall safety goggles and face shields the provide droplet and splash protection.

Another important step is making sure to have running water available to wash your eyes, if you need it. I haven't had running water in my studio space in years, so I always make sure to have an eyewash station setup and ready to go.

Keeping Your Skin Safe

Soapmaking is hands-on, so it makes sense to protect your hands! All soapmakers should wear gloves that can withstand exposure to lye solution, raw soap, and fragrance materials. I personally prefer nitrile gloves, as I'm allergic to latex. They come in a variety of lengths, so you can get more forearm coverage, if you wish. My favorite thing about nitrile gloves is that they are used in a variety of professions, so there are a ton of sizing options out there.

Some soapmakers use dishwashing gloves. Unfortunately, dishwashing gloves tend to be bulky which can hinder your dexterity (and most are made of latex!)

Other Skin Protection Measures

Some soapmakers also wear long sleeves, an apron, and/or a labcoat to protect their skin and clothing. If you choose to wear long sleeves or any other skin protection, ensure that it's either waterproof or can be removed easily. When wearing long sleeves, a splash of lye solution will soak into the fabric and sit on your skin. In order to rinse your skin and dilute the lye solution for removal, you need to remove the fabric as well.

Breathing Clean Air

A lot of soapmakers are aware of the dangers of mixing lye solution and the resulting kickback of particles and fumes. The most common precaution most soapmakers follow is either mixing lye solution outside or under an exhaust hood in a kitchen. A sudden change in wind direction outside can completely negate any attempt at safety outside, and an exhaust hood in a kitchen is not likely designed to extract caustic particles!

While mixing lye solution can be disastrous for your respiratory system, soapmakers often forget that essential oils, fragrance oils, and colorant particles are also in the air we breathe. All of these ingredients hang out in the air long after you've made a batch of soap, especially as soap sits on a shelf and cures for weeks at a time in your space.

Wear a Respirator

I highly recommend snagging and wearing a respirator while making soap. You want a respirator with replaceable cartridges that filter both particulate and volatile organic compounds. Some filters are rendered ineffective by oil droplets in the air, so it's important to check which filters are compatible with the ingredients you are using. The upside to using a respirator is that full face shield respirators are available, which kills two birds with one stone!

Keeping the Air in Your Space Clean

Besides using a respirator, you should consider a fan exhaust system or fume extractor in your space to help clean the air regularly, both during making and curing of your soap. Before using a fan exhaust or installing one, make sure to check with your local environmental regulations to make sure you don't need to use a specific kind of filter or if you need a certain kind of system.

If you have a studio space that doesn't accommodate installation of a system, an air purifier can help clean the air (but is not typically enough on its own.) In my current studio space, I'm not able to install a fan exhaust or fume extractor, so an air purifier is better than nothing at all. Again, you need to remember that you likely are dealing with both particulate and VOCs, so keep that in mind when choosing an air purifier.

Having Emergency Backup On Hand

Most safety practices are active means of protection, like wearing personal protective gear and being respectful of the ingredients you are using. However, having proactive safety measures in place can also be a lifesaver.

I don't know a single soapmaker who hasn't experienced some kind of accidental spill, whether it's tipping a soap pot or lye solution container, spilling oils, or dropping glass fragrance bottles! Being clumsy, I've done it all. From spilling 35 pounds of castor oil on my studio floor to dropping full 16 ounce glass bottle of essential oil and more, being prepared for spills has saved my hide on numerous occasions.

Be Prepared for Spills

For oil or water spills, a basic granular absorbent is necessary to have on hand. (In a pinch, a giant bag of clay cat litter also works. Ask me how I know…) For hobbyist soapmakers who don't have a lot of ingredients on hand, a small bag or container of absorbent or portable universal spill kit will work just fine. For production soapmakers, larger spill kits for each ingredient type are necessary. To determine how big of a spill kit you need, evaluate the maximum size of an ingredient you may work with, whether it's a drum of oils or a five gallon bucket of lye solution, and the type of ingredient (oil, water, hazmat, etc.)

Keep Information at Your Fingertips

You also want to keep all safety information on hand and easy to access. I personally keep a binder of Safety Data Sheets for every ingredient on hand, organized alphabetically, so I can easily find information about an ingredient if needed. I also recommend having a contact list on hand for any needs, such as poison control, hazardous waste disposal, emergency personnel, medical contacts, etc.

Creating A Plan & Following A Process

Over time, all soapmakers develop a flow to their soapmaking process that actually helps them make handmade soap safely. How so? When you always follow a specific protocol, you prevent mistakes and find issues before they blow up in your face.

Personally, I like to prep everything before I get started. Here's the order in which I flow:

Make my lye solution (or weigh my premixed lye solution)

Weigh and melt my soaping oils (or weigh my masterbatched oils)

Weigh and add my fragrance to my soaping oils (so I can't forget to add it later)

Measure and premix my colorants (in measuring cups big enough for the soap to be added)

Check my measurements and prepped ingredients against my formula

Clean my work surface (to give me a completely clear area to work in)

Lay out my ingredients for the batch to my left, and my mold or any swirling/texturing tools to the right

As each ingredient is added to the soap pot, I move the empty container to the right (so when I'm all done, there should be nothing to the left)

Double check my formula against the empty containers, and the total soap weight in the mold versus the formula

This process prevents me from forgetting anything in my formula, as well as minimizing spills or mishaps because there is a specific order and flow. There's two steps that require me to double check what I'm doing to make sure everything is accurate and precise.

Keep Records of Your Batches

In addition to developing a flow to your soapmaking process, keeping top notch records will also help you make handmade soap safely. For every batch of soap you make, there should be a record of the ingredients used, the date it was made, and how long it was cured.

For hobbyists, I recommend printing out your formula from SoapCalc or Soapmaker 3 and putting it in a plastic sheet protector before making the soap. Then you can use a dry erase marker to make any notes or adjustments, as well as check off ingredients as you go. When you are finished, you can print a modified formula based on your notes, put the date on it, and then place it in a three ring binder that compiles all of your "made batches" into a recording system.

If the batch doesn't turn out right, or something goes wrong, you have the tools at your disposal to learn from it right away! As an added bonus to the practice, it will get you in the habit of proper record keeping should you ever decide to start a business.

Have a Plan for Safety

Another proactive planning step you should take is creating safety plans which dictate how you fix or handle a problem. You should have a plan for:

- How to determine if your handmade soap is safe to use

- How to clean up a spill of each ingredient type

- What to do with soap that is lye heavy, oil heavy, heavily fragranced, etc.

Make sure to write each plan out step by step. Have your spill plan posted in a visible place in your soapmaking area. You never know what might happen, whether or not you will be present to clean up the spill, or if you might be injured and unable to clean it up. It's a good idea to indicate where you keep your Safety Data Sheets in the spill clean up plan, too!

CHAPTER THREE

CHOOSE THE RIGHT SOAPMAKING EqUIPMENT

Soap-making can be a fun and rewarding hobby, its also essential to have a good soap making guide as it can also be dangerous if the soap-maker doesn't research their materials, and take the proper precautions when making soap.

Lye is caustic and corrosive, meaning that it burns like acid when it comes into contact with skin or other surfaces.

Vinegar can help to neutralize lye when it is spilled, and prevent it from damaging surfaces, so it is a good idea to keep some on hand when working with lye.

Also, protect your work area with plastic bags, newspaper, or a vinyl tablecloth; make sure your work space is well-ventilated, because lye tends to evaporate quickly, and releases toxic fumes when it mixes with water. (If at all possible, it's best to make soap outside, so that spills and ventilation are non issues.)

Keep children and pets away from your work area and materials, and be sure to clean your equipment after each use; store lye properly in a tightly-sealed container, out of the reach of children and pets.

During the soap-making and cleanup process, be sure to wear protective equipment, in case you spill the lye on yourself.

A long-sleeve shirt, long pants, socks and shoes are all absolutely necessary.

You'll also want to don safety goggles, heavy-duty rubber gloves (or latex dishwashing gloves), and a rubber or latex apron; the more protection you have from lye spills or splashes, the better.

Make sure that the rest of the equipment you plan to use - containers, mixers, etc. - is safe for use with lye.

Lye reacts adversely with some materials, such as copper or aluminum, so all containers should be made of glass, stainless steel, enamel, or plastic.

Your equipment list should include, but is not limited to, the following:

- Two sturdy plastic half-gallon pitchers - one for water, one for lye.
- Large heat-resistant container, for mixing the lye and water.
- Large stainless steel mixing bowl - should be large enough to accommodate lye, water and oils, without overflow or splatter.
- Small glass or plastic containers, for holding oils after they are measured and before they are mixed together.

- Two sturdy plastic stirring spoons - one for the lye-water mixture, one for the oils.

- Two glass candy thermometers - one for the lye-water mixture, one for the oils.

- Large (16-qt.) enameled or stainless steel pot, for heating oils.

- Old blanket, for insulating soap molds.

- Kitchen scale or postal scale, accurate to 1 gram or 0.1 ounces.

- Plastic cling wrap or wax paper, for lining soap molds.

- Soap molds - can be anything you like, from elaborate plastic candy molds to wooden boxes to milk cartons or capped PVC pipe sections.

- Stick blender - optional, but will create a much faster trace.

- Pot holders/oven mitts.

- Plastic spatula, to scrape soap batter out of mixing bowl and into molds.

Make sure you have all of your equipment assembled and ready to go before you begin the soap-making process; you can ruin a large batch of batter by stopping to look for something, or run to the store.

An important part of the soap-making process is timing, and materials will continue to cool, and saponification will continue to take place, with or without you being there.

Be sure to clean your materials when you are done, use them only for soap-making, and keep them all together for the sake of convenience.

Here is a list of the all-important tools of the trade. Please select those that are applicable for the method of soap making you will be employing.

Long sleeved shirt or lab coat to protect your arms from potential splashes.

Rubber gloves to protect your hands from the caustic solution and mixture

Goggles or some kind of protective eye wear to protect the obvious - your eyes. (Regular glasses do not count by themselves). Face shields work great.

Face masks preferably with a filter to guard against inhaling the caustic fumes from your lye solution.

Long pants and some kind of footwear to protect your feet from spills.

At least 2 sturdy plastic, stainless steel or glass containers. One for measuring your lye (sodium hydroxide) crystals, one for measuring your liquid.

A minimum of 2 sturdy plastic or stainless steel spoons for stirring the lye solution and the oils.

Glass candy or candle/soap making thermometers.

Plastic buckets or large stainless steel saucepans/pots for heating and mixing the soap mixture in.

Newspapers, old blankets, quilts or sheets to help protect your counter space if you do not have a designated soap making area.

Freezer paper, parchment paper, saran wrap or even sheets of plastic or plastic bags for lining your molds. (of course, this will depend on the type of mold you will be using. If you will be using bar soap molds like the Milky Way type, then you will need a can of baking spray like Pam for easy release of the soap from the mold.

Kitchen scale - perfect for the hobby soap maker, if possible try to obtain an electronic scale for more accurate measurements.

Spice/coffee grinder - perfect for grinding herbs and other additives to incorporate into your recipe.

Hand grater - great for melt and pour soap making, as well as rebatching soap.

Molds of choice - can be anything from drawer liners (Rubber Maid type), to plastic bar or tray molds, or even wooden molds. Plastic food storage containers work as well.

Stick Blender - very useful for achieving a faster trace in cold process soap making.

Rubber Spatulas - useful for getting that last bit of soap mixture out of your mixing container.

Small glass or plastic containers to hold herbs, fragrance/essential oils, colorants or other additives until you are ready to use them.

Paper towels or other pieces of cloth to help clean up spills as they occur.

Now that you have got your tools together - happy soaping. Do not forget to always prepare your work area before you start. There is nothing worst than having started your soap making process only to realize you do not have all the tools and equipment you need.

The only tools you need are commonly found in kitchens such as:

Accurate scale

The scale must be in good order, meaning it measures with absolute accuracy. Whenever possible choose a scale that can weigh as low as 1/10th of an ounce. Precision is important in making soap and all your ingredients like oils, lye, fragrance, and additives even water must be measured properly.

Safety goggles and rubber gloves

These are important to keep you away from harm, especially your eyes and hands. Lye solutions may cause harm as well as the caustic raw materials.

Heat resistant plastic or stainless pitcher with lid

A two to three quart heat resistant plastic is used for mixing lye solution. If possible label it with "lye solution - be careful".

Plastic or stainless spoon

A plastic spoon or stainless may be used in stirring the lye solution.

A large pyrex pitcher may be used in making soap in small batches about two to three pounds. For bigger batches of soap, a steel pot is preferred about eight to twelve quarts in size. This can also be use for melting oils and blending the soap. Do not forget to use a pot with a lid.

Plastic or glass bowl or pitcher

Use a two to three quarts plastic or glass bowl to measure and hold liquid oils before pouring or adding to the soap pot. Large bowls may also be used.

Ramekins, beakers, and measuring cups

This are soap making equipment used to hold fragrance oils, essential oils, colorants, separated soaps, and additives. These are set aside while waiting to be poured on the soap pots.

Spoons and whisks

Spoons and whisks are used to blend or mix colorants, fragrance oils and other melted oils before pouring to the soap.

Stainless or plastic ladle

Used to ladle out a little soap mixture to blend colorants, providing color to the soap.

Stick Blender

From the name itself these are used to blend oils with the lye mixture which is the start of the saponification process.

Soap Mold

Soap mold is the final appearance of your soap. This is where the raw soap is poured. Molds can be in any form and any leak-proof container that is made of plastic, glass, or stainless steel.

Rubber spatulas

Used to completely scrape all soap solution from the pot.

Paper Towels

To wipe off spills and cover the soap in the mold to retain heat.

Soap making equipment is indeed readily available in one's kitchen or any area in the house. All you need to do is to look around, collect the tools needed, set them aside whilst you prepare the area where the soap making process is done. Tools may be added according to the needs that may arise as you get to exercise the process of soap making.

CHAPTER FOUR

THE IMPORTANCE THINGS TO KNOW ABOUT SOAP MAKING

Soap making enthusiasts have been increasing in numbers over the years. If you just learned about this through the internet or through friends I would gladly say that you should try it. You will be amazed how wonderful and rewarding soap making can be. You do not only need to know the process but also what soap making supply you need.

The supplies you need are the basic ingredients you need in making them. Therefore it is important to be acquainted with the ingredients and learn about its characteristics and functions. You need soap making supplies like lye, fragrance oils, basic oils, equipments and molds.

I will share to you the basic supplies you need:

1. Safety devices - you will need rubber gloves and goggles to protect your skin & eyes from burns. This is the very first thing you need before starting the process even in preparation time.

2. Weighing scale - you need a weighing scale that shows measurements in grams and in ounces. Soap making requires accuracy in

measuring ingredients, therefore it is vital to have one.

3. Containers - the containers you need are not just any container, it should be heat resistant. Have a three-quarter size or bigger depending on your need.

4. Stainless pots - Use only large stainless pots when mixing the lye, basic oils or fats and fragrance oils.

5. Stainless sauce pans - Basically a three-quart stainless sauce pan is used for heating the solid ingredients oils, fats and additives.

6. Silicone Utensils - Use only this type of utensil when mixing your ingredients or any other soap solutions. Wood on the other hand will tend to corrode when it comes in contact with lye and breaks which in the long run makes it expensive because you need to repurchase again. That is why I highly recommend the use of silicone utensils.

7. Thermometers - You need this in measuring lye and oil temperatures.

8. Soap molds - you can be creative when choosing your soap molds. You can buy or make your own soap whichever you want as long as it is suitable with the kind of soap you are making. What is important is to determine how often you are going to use your mold. If you are making soaps only for your family

then you can use any soap molds. But if you are planning to make soap making a business, I suggest you buy quality molds available in reputable stores.

9. Wax Paper - you need to place wax paper in your molds for ease of removing your soap bars from its mold and to cover your finished products to preserve heat from dispersing so fast. You may buy any brand of wax paper in the supermarket.

10. Tapes - this is used to keep wax paper in place.

11. Soap cutter - this are optional soap equipment. If you are only making soaps for the family, you may use kitchen knife instead. But if you are cutting soap for selling purposes then a soap cutter is required for finer and clean edges.

12. Fragrance oils and other additives - These are optional as well. If you want your soap to have additives like essential oils or scents then you just buy the particular oil you want. But of course you need to follow precautionary steps, use oils that are compatible with your other ingredients and that blends well with an organic soap making supply.

CHAPTER FIVE

HOW TO BLEND ESSENTIAL OILS FOR NATURAL BEAUTY AND SOAP MAKING

In the process of soap or cosmetic making, many essential oils are blended together to give women the natural beauty she craves for. This whole process itself requires considerable skill and talent as different kinds of fragrances as well as products having medicinal properties have to be blended in certain prescribed proportion only. On many occasions, different blends require many trials even before they are finalized.

The essential oils that make the blends are floral, resin, earthy, spicy, citrus, medicinal or herbaceous oils. Essential oils are characterized on the basis of their aromatic effects-top note, middle note as well as bottom/base note.

Once classification is established and learned it will be much easier to blend different scents and oil properties. But their are some things you should know before you start the blending process.

First, it is very important to make sure that your oils are pure and fresh. It is also important to make sure you are using the appropriate oil because each oil has different requirements and necessities associated with it. The oil should be pure as well as of good quality, and not fragrance oil (fragrance oils are much different than essential oils). You also require small glass bottles with tight caps, diffusers as well as carrier oils. To start with you can make use of the floral oils; these oils can be blended very easily and also give the results we long cherish. You can blend floral oils with citrus, spicy as well as woodsy oils. These woodsy oils can easily get blended with different kinds of oils in different categories.

Besides it is suggested not to have many blends constituting spicy and citrus oils, as they can cause difficulty in blending and also don't give that aromatic effect as we desire. It is also important to know that while blending, oils are to be added in drops to ensure not to have more than requisite blending. Ratio of blending is 30-35 per cent for the top note, between 40-50 per cent for middle note, and bottom/base note in the quantity of 20-25 per cent.

For diluting a mixture, a general ratio for 1 tablespoon of your desired carrier oil is 2 to 5 drops of essential oils. Once they are ready, you need to store it in tightly capped bottle preventing any kind of contamination, mishandling as well as leaking. If blend is very strong then it is all the more necessary to add some quantity of carrier oil to the mixture for diluting your natural beauty product or soap a little.

There might be some occasions where you will find

certain blends smelling wonderfully while some very medicinal, spicy or too strong. It is better to note down each essential oil blend as it will help you in recreating the blend in future.

Tips to Using Essential and Fragile Oils When Making Soap

When making soap, it can be very frustrating to use your favorite oils for fragrance only to have them "burn off" before you've even had a chance to pour the soap into a mold. Not to mention, some of these fragrances can be a bit too pricey to just be throwing away! In this article you will discover how to use these oils when making soap in a way that holds their integrity.

First, it's important to understand that essential oils(EO) and fragile oils are not necessarily the same. Although many essential oils are considered fragile, there are some which have a much higher flash point (evaporating temperature) than others. Still, it is best to follow these tips with any essential oils you use to be safe.

Use cold process soap making.

As a soap maker, I have always had trouble with hot process soap making and EO. I therefore recommend that you use cold process soap making if you plan to use essential oils. When you use cold process, make sure your melted hard oils and lye/water mixture hover around 100 - 120 degrees before mixing them together. To accomplish this you will most likely need to use 1 or 2 ice baths.

Do not add the essential oils too early.

When making soap, it is vital not to add your oils and herbs too early. For this reason, soap makers wait until after they've blended their soap to the point of trace. After reaching trace you can add your EOs and any herbs you might be using. Doing it before almost always guarantees that they will be ruined - and your soap might be, too!

Mix fragile oils with carrier oils.

Almost all soap recipes call for a fairly large quantity of carrier oils to provide the fat necessary for saponification. These "carrier oils" include Olive, Palm Kernel, Coconut, etc and these oils have a much higher flash point than almost all essential oils. A trick I learned years ago was to measure out the carrier oils, then take out about 1 teaspoon from that measurement and add it to your mix of EOs. Obviously, the exact amount depends on the size of your soap batch and amount of essential oils, but 1 teaspoon seems to work most times. Mix the carrier oil with your essential oils to sort of strengthen them, then add them after trace.

These three tips will help you use EOs when making soap without all that frustration and waste. New soap makers may also find it helpful to find more advice on the web or from instructional books and videos. Soap making is very easy once you get the hang of it, but getting the hang of it can be a bit frustrating if you have no one to help you!

Scenting Your

Scenting handmade soaps is a matter of personal preference.

There are two varieties of oils that can be used to scent soap: fragrance oils, and essential oils. Either can be used, according to the preferences of the soap-maker.

Fragrance oils are made from a mixture of aroma chemicals. They are commonly used when there is no essential oil available for a particular fragrance, or when the essential oil is far too costly, or environmentally irresponsible, to use. Unlike essential type oils, fragrance oils can be part natural and part synthetic, or all synthetic.

Fragrance oils are usually thinned with diluents, to help thin out the compounds and create some uniformity of pungency across the spectrum of fragrance oils that are available.

Essential type oils, on the other hand, are all-natural fragrances that are taken from various plants and herbs. The oil can come from any part of a plant, but are most often taken from the flowers and leaves. Many essential type oils are associated with a particular benefit or effect, and they are often used in aromatherapy. It takes many (sometimes thousands) of pounds of a plant to make a pound of essential oil; because of this, pure essential type oils are much more expensive than fragrance oils.

Deciding which one to use is a matter of preference, and can depend on a variety of factors. If cost is an issue, fragrance oils might be a better option than essential oils; as with most things, there are different grades, and the better ones tend to be more expensive.

There are some well-known scents can only be found in fragrance oils, because there are no natural blends to match them. The cons of fragrance oils are that they don't tend to last as long as essential oils, because they are diluted, and the alcohol in them evaporates quickly.

Pure essential oils are undiluted, so they tend to be stronger, and last longer in soap. There are some scents that can only be found in these oils, and simply cannot be mimicked by synthetic compounds. Essential oils are also easier for amateur soap-makers to use, because the additives in fragrance oils make the soap batter prone to seizing.

Essential oils made from plants that have beneficial

effects are known to retain those effects, and pass them on to your soap, as well; however, if you want your essential oils to retain the vitamins and antioxidants they possess before soap-making, it is best to use the cold-process method, and add them at trace - the heat from the hot-process method can break down these nutrients, and destroy their ability to nourish your skin.

Another problem with essential oils is that they are volatile, and while they are long-lasting in soap, they evaporate □ uickly when exposed to air, so the process of mixing them into the soap must be expeditious.

As previously stated, there are pros and cons to both oils, and which product you use to scent your soap will be a matter of personal preference.

As with all other aspects of the soap-making process, learn as much as you can about the fragrance or essential oils you plan to use, so that you can make an educated decision about which one to utilize for your soap.

Also, regardless of which one you choose, make sure that it has been tested and proven safe for use in soap-making, and if you are making soap for someone you know, you may want to do a test to see if the intended recipient is allergic to the substance.

Beginners Guide To Soap Making

Making your own soap is a lot of fun. I love making my own soap for myself and also giving it as gifts to family and friends. If you're interested in making your own soap but not sure where to start, here's a brief explanation of the three different soap making processes:

Cold Process

Cold process soap making is really making soap from scratch. The three basic ingredients you'll need to make soap this way are water, oils and sodium hydroxide (lye). Lye is classed as a hazardous material. It can burn skin on contact. When using lye you need to be extremely careful and take all safety precautions, such as wearing safety goggles, protective gloves, clothing and shoes. You also need to ensure you use a stainless steel saucepan and have separate containers for the storing of lye and measuring cups, etc just for soap making.

It's very important you use a good recipe if making soap this way that tells you all the precautions you need to take when using lye; such as mixing the water and lye outside or in a very well ventilated area. The mixing of water and lye first produces a steam so toxic that it can burn your lungs.

You need to be very responsible when handling lye and it does sound scary, so a lot of soap making beginners prefer starting off making their own soap by the following two methods.

Handmilled or Rebatched Method

This method involves the grating of ready made soap (so there's no lye to worry about) that is then melted with added water. You can add your own additives, such as flower petals, herbs, lavender, oatmeal, spices, soap colors and fragrance. Then you pour it into soap molds and leave to set. This can take 24 hours but for a truly hardened soap it can take up to two weeks.

Melt and Pour Method

In my experience, this is the easiest method to use if you're a beginner. Melt and pour soap comes in ready made soap blocks (no lye to deal with). You just melt it, either in the microwave or double boiler, add your soap color, fragrance and optional additives, pour it into the mold and leave it to set for a few hours. Once it's set it's ready to use!

When making soap by any of the methods above, it's important you use a good recipe so you get the measurements of the soap, colourings, fragrances and additives right. It's also important that you don't accidentally splash yourself when dealing with a hot, melted soap mixture.

Soap making is addictive. Once you make your first successful batch, you don't want to stop! So why not get started on your soap making journey today?

CHAPTER SIX

HOW TO MAKE LIQUID SOAP

For those familiar with cold process soap making, the lye solution uses sodium hydroxide (NaOH) for saponification to produce bar soap. If you want to learn how to make liquid soap, the first thing you need to know is that liquid soap does not involve this type of lye. Instead, to make liquid soap you will need potassium hydroxide (KOH), known as potash lye. Both of these types of lye are extremely caustic and will burn your skin, so extreme care must be taking when you're learning how to make soap.

Before you attempt to make liquid soap, it is a good idea to familiarize yourself with the cold process of soap making first. Beginners will find it more difficult to try to make liquid soap first, as it is a bit more complicated and requires a great deal of patience as well as a bit of extra time!

Similar to the cold process in that the lye mixture and fats are blended, liquid soap requires a lot of blending but instead uses heat to saponify the liquid. Reaching trace is a lengthy stirring process; to make liquid soap you will need to keep stirring or blending for about 30 minutes so a stick blender is a must if you want to know how to make liquid soap without getting cramp in your arm! Once the mixture reaches trace, the next stage is a waiting game. With an occasional stir every half hour or so, the soap will take up to 4 hours to cook, and its state will change several times throughout this period.

The next stage in your quest to make liquid soap is to test the soap mixture, to make sure it will stay clear. If all is well, water is added to dilute the "gloppy" mixture, but it is not quite ready yet to turn into liquid soap consistency you have been hoping to make! After several rounds of waiting and stirring, the paste will eventually dissolve and you'll be ready to neutralize the liquid soap mixture. This process involves adding boric acid, and is required to get rid of the excess lye that is involved when you make liquid soap.

To make liquid soap smell pleasant, you will now need to add essential oils or fragrance to the mixture, and if you'd like a bit of color in your liquid soap, a coloring additive can also be used. Leave the liquid soap to cool and pour it into large containers to rest.

Now that you know how to make liquid soap, you are ready to divide up your mixture into individual containers, bottles or dispensing jars. Your soap is now ready to place in your bathroom and use for washing hands, as shower wash or shampoo, depending on the recipe you have used to make your liquid soap.

Marie Ackland - Soap making was originally a hobby of mine that gave me great pleasure, theres something quite satisfying about creating from scratch a beautifully scented bar of soap.

It then turned into a full time passion, creating wonderful soap for family and friends to enjoy. When a friend surgested I take some along to a local craft fair, which I did and from that day on I never looked back. I now have a great soap business which makes a healthy profit and gives me great satisfaction.

Melt And Pour Process

As you will learn, soap making can be simple or complex. Some people enjoy the challenge of going all out professionally, which is fine. However, other people simply want to make soap for personal use or to give as an occasional gift.

Keep in mind that safety precautions should still be followed because soap becomes dangerously hot when melted, regardless of the skill level involved. Here, we will discuss easy melt and pour techniques, perfect for the novice or skilled soap maker!

First, keep in mind that most handmade soap is made from glycerin. When you purchase store-bought soap, the majority of the glycerin has been processed out. Therefore, when you make your own soap, you have a great opportunity to create something that is glycerin rich and soft.

Although "glycerin" is usually clear, with today's colors and fragrances, you can create beautiful soaps that not only make your skin soft but also look great. With glycerin, because it is a humectant, moisture is drawn out of itself. That means when you use glycerin soap while bathing, a very fine layer will stay on the skin, adding moisture.

Buying Soap

To go through the easy melt and pour method, you want to stop by your soap-making supply or hobby store, or online soap supply store. There, you will find large blocks of clear soap. These vary in size and type. Remember, the prices will vary depending on where you live and the store or business where you buy.

Regardless, the following are the types of melt and pour soaps you would need to make your homemade soap.

Hemp Glycerin Soap

This type of glycerin is great for the "melt and pour" system, creating semi transparent soap with the benefit of hemp. Hemp oil is rich with essential fatty acids, enzymes, Omega 3 and 6, and vitamins A, D, & E. When buying hemp glycerin, you should look for blocks that are around 20% glycerin, is alcohol free, and free of any harsh detergents.

Typically, you will find 11-pound slabs, which will make approximately 44 bars of soap, each four ounces. If that is too much, you might try to find smaller slabs or go in with another soap maker to split the soap. This size slab will average $40.

Olive Oil Soap

Olive oil soap is semi-transparent with just a slight tan color. However, the benefits and features are very close to that of hemp glycerin. The only difference is that instead of hemp, olive oil is used. When buying, look for cold pressed olive oil that contains essential fatty acids, minerals, vitamins, and as close to 20% glycerin as possible. Again, an 11-pound slab for olive oil soap runs around $40.

Clear Glycerin Soap

This type of soap is transparent and has low shrinkage qualities. In addition, clear glycerin soap has very little problem with discoloration. This soap is vegetable derived and an excellent choice for "melt and pour" soap bars. You can add color or fragrance easily and the soap will leave your skin feeling soft and smooth.

Clear glycerin soap is also a great choice for making soap with multiple layers, novelty soaps (those with toys, flowers, or other objects inside), and yet the clarity is exactly what you would buy from your favorite boutique. If you want a good daily soap, one that is fun for the kids, and makes an excellent gift, clear glycerin is it.

Goat's Milk Glycerin Soap

This type of soap originates from the beautiful Rocky Mountains. The feel is creamy and rich, and very luxurious. The appearance of this soap is off white. Many people shy away from goat's milk glycerin because of the name but you will find that it has no fragrance and actually takes both color and fragrance perfectly.

If you want soap that is natural, this is a great choice. Typically, goat's milk glycerin soap is slightly higher than the other types of soaps but still very affordable and well worth the investment.

Melt And Pour Soap Making Equipment And Ingredients

The great thing about using melt and pour is that you can use equipment you typically have on hand. With this method, you can use the base of a double boiler or your microwave oven.

Keep in mind that if you choose the microwave, the bowl with the soap substance will need to be covered with plastic wrap to keep it from splattering but more importantly, to help keep the excess moisture from evaporating. For the microwave method, you would melt the base soap on high for about one minute, stirring in the remaining pieces not yet melted.

For the double boiler option, bring the water to a boil. Then, add your melt and pour soap of choice, cover, and leave on low. This will take quite some time to melt so about every 10 minutes, check the base to see if it is melted. If you like, you can stir occasionally to ensure an even melt.

Fragrance

For both methods of melt and pour, if you want to add in fragrance, once the base soap has melted, then you would add the fragrance oil. Be sure the fragrance is mixed in completely and that the base of the soap does not have a cloudy appearance.

Although you can use more or less fragrance according to personal preference, typically a good rule to follow is to use .25 ounces to every one pound of soap base. In addition to fragrances, you can also use essential oils.

Color

Now for the color, if you want to create colored soap, add approximately one-eighth teaspoon to one-quarter teaspoon mica in with the melting soap base, making sure to mix in it well.

If any bubbles form on top of the soap, you can leave them for design effect or spray them with rubbing alcohol. If you want to use food coloring, start with just one drop to the melted base, stirring well. Then, you can add one additional drop until you find the color of preference.

After the fragrance and color have been added to the soap base, pour the melted base into the mold of your choice. Again, if you want to remove any bubbles that will settle on top, spray them with rubbing alcohol. After the soap has hardened, generally a few hours, you can use it and enjoy!

Cost

As you can see, to make your own soap at home, you would pay around $40 for the slab of base, a few dollars for fragrance, a few dollars for coloring, and that is about it. The process is very cost effective, fun, and you end up with exactly the type of soap you love most.

Most people figure that one bar of homemade soap will average .50, far less than you would pay elsewhere. In addition, you can add in special items or effects to jazz things up.

Making soap using the melt and pour process is easy and fun... and makes for very inexpensive soap. Not only is it great for making your own soap, but it makes for truly unique and creative gifts.

Essential Oils For Aromatherapy in Handmade Bath Products

Aromatic herbs and oils have been used since ancient times in religious rites, for perfumes, cosmetics, and for therapeutic and medicinal purposes. Written records documenting various uses of herbs and essential oils made from herbs, go back as far as four thousand years. Ancient India, ancient Egypt, ancient Greece and Rome all document the usage of aromatic herbs and oils.

The modern practice of aromatherapy was introduced in the late 1920's, when Rene-Maurice Gattefosse discovered the healing properties of lavender. He noticed that lavender oil, when applied to a burn on his hand, seemed to heal the wound quickly and later thought that it reduced scaring. He then became interested in the therapeutic uses of essential oils. Gattefosse concluded that natural oils were more effective than artificially produced synthetics.

Dr. Jean Valnet treated psychiatric patients in a program using essential oils and published his results in 1964, calling the therapy 'Aromatherapie'.

The word, aromatherapy, may be construed to mean that they scent itself is the primary source of healing.

But it is more than just fragrance. Essential oils penetrate the skin and influence body chemistry, as we see in the use of oils in massage. For instance, if garlic oil is rubbed on the soles of your feet, a garlic odor will appear on your breath some time later.

So, aromatherapy has several avenues of affecting a person.

Using natural oils in your bath a few drops sprinkles in the tub, mixed with various bath products and lotions, or added to soap can effect your mood with its scent. Various oils can also be useful to heal wounds, skin irritations, rashes, and insect bites. Certain oils are effective insect repellants. Some can aid in the treatment of acne and fungal conditions, while others help oily skin or act as moisturizers for dry skin.

Essential oils are often used in home made bath products such a bath salt combinations and hand made soaps. It is a good idea to test for skin sensitivity before committing yourself to creating a whole batch of home made product using essential oils. If you use essential oils at home, check for toxic properties of the oils that interest you.

You can research and learn which oils would benefit your skin type or special skin conditions. Learn which ones are beneficial to mood enhancement. Some oils are stimulants while others encourage relaxation. A stimulating oil like peppermints better to used in the shower before work, while a relaxing one, like valerian is best used for a soothing bath before bed.

Learn how to blend essential oils to create unique fragrances. The proper combination of scents make for long lasting, pleasant aromas. Blending oils that do not go well together can lead to a product that does not smell good or an aroma that does not have staying power.

Essential oils can be purchased through herbalists, at specialty shops, ethnic groceries, or online. Shop around when looking for these wonderful oils. Essential oils can be very expensive and there is a wide discrepancy between pricing. Just remember, when you buy oils, purchase natural essential oils and not the artificial fragrance oils. While the synthetics may smell nice, they do not have the lasting power that essential oils do, and they do not have the therapeutic properties that can improve your skin.

More often than we realize, people are drawn to a soap or are encouraged to buy soap because of the way it smells. In fact, most big companies know that the scent of a soap plays a large role in the success of a product. Scent is a factor that can make or break a product, which is why getting it right is almost as important as getting the soap blend right. No one will buy a soap that has fabulous skin benefits, but gives them a headache!

The scents of most soaps are reliant on the fragrance oils or the essential oils used in the soap. Fragrance oils are often synthetic, which is less than ideal for those who want all natural soap. Essential oils, on the other hand, are made from plant extracts and are completely natural, however they are far more potent and can give the soap certain properties. Soaps made with these oils are soaps carry the fragrance of the oil, but the essences are also a way to enhance the soap's characteristics.

Essential oils are commonly used to give a soap therapeutic properties, specifically aromatherapy. The scent of these oils can calm, invigorate, relax, and soothe a person while they enjoy their bath. Oils are also often used to give the soap a property that will add to the benefits of the consumer. For example, tea tree oil, which carries anti-bacterial properties can help make a soap naturally anti-bacterial. It can also make the soap ideal for treating acne.

There are many different types of essential oils for soap making, which leads to many different types of soap. However, one must be careful when working with these oils because can be volatile, so they should be kept away from heat and should always be sealed properly. Very expensive oils should be kept in a refrigerator. Not only will this make it last longer, but it is also likely to be expensive because it is pure.

Apart from being volatile, these oils are also very

potent. This means you should ideally use gloves while mixing them and wash your hands after each use. It is important not to get any in your eyes, and if you do, to wash your eyes right away. When mixing, be sure to mix in small batches and to always mix the essential oils with a fixed oil. This will make sure your mixture is not overpowering, and also ensure that your final product is safe for the skin.

Essential oils are often added before a soap mixture reaches trace. Each batch of soap will only need a few drops of oil. Apart from making sure the scents blend well, it is also important to make sure the oils do not have a negative effect on the soap, as it can sometimes have when mixed with certain ingredients. In order to prevent waste, make some trial batches and monitor the soap to see how well it reacts. When unsure, study the various soap making recipes and see how oils are blended into soap and in what amounts. This should give you a decent guide on how to use these oils.

Herbal Soap Making

What is herbal soap? They are soaps that are mixed with natural ingredients such as juice, extract, or even chopped leaves of herbal plants. Herbal are safe to use except for those excessively sensitive skin, they should be vigilant for herbs that may irritate them.

Making herbal soaps are generally similar with other soap making process, what makes them distinctive to other process is the adding and choice of herbs incorporated into the soap. What are the herbs that are best used in soaps? Mint is a good choice for everyday soap that gives the user that invigorating effect while lavender is best for a soothing fragrance that a lady may desire. For herbs that provide the whitening effect on the skin, choose herbs such as papaya, kalamansi, or kamias.

Guava and akapulko may give the medicinal benefits for anti-fungal or antiseptic properties. Avocado and cucumber are one of the best herbal beauty soaps. Once the herbs to be used are selected it is time to start making your first ever herbal soap.

Choose the herbs that you want, more so, combining different herbs helps in producing something different and something unique. Experimenting is the key to a new found soap combination which is what herbal soap making is all about. It is quite challenging but also exciting to do.

The soap making procedure:

1. Prepare 1/4 cups of water and bring to a boil and add the herb of your choice, about 2 tablespoons of finely ground herbs. Let it steep for fifteen minutes.

2. Pour in the steeped mixture into a double boiler then reheat.

3. Add the soap which has already been cut into

pieces and melt. Coloring and essential oils may also be added at this time to make your soap more attractive.

4. Once the mixture and the soap have completely mixed and totally melted, pour the soap into the mold and let it harden at room temperature. Coat the mold with vegetable oil before pouring the mixture in order to remove soap from mold easily.

5. After a few hours check if the soap has already hardened and remove from the mold.

6. Do not use the soap yet, let it cure for another day or two.

Herbal soap making is so simple, with the proper herbs and the skill to make the soap and presto...your new handcrafted soap!

Why is it that a lot of women and even men are gaga about herbal soap making? If you have not tried herbal soaps then you are doing your skin an injustice. Just taking a harmless bath once or twice daily may be damaging to your skin because the soap you are using may contain chemicals that are harsh to your skin. Soaps with synthetic chemicals strips the skin of its protective oils and may cause dryness, flaking and skin dehydration.

Herbal soap is the answer to some of your skin problems because it helps to moisturize your skin and preserve the skin's smoothness and suppleness. Making and using your own herbal soap has a lot of advantages for you and, who knows, it may be your key to a youthful skin.

No preservatives. Homemade herbal soaps have no preservatives thus it does not contain any ingredients that can irritate the skin. In fact, these soaps can be used by babies because you are sure that they are 100% all natural.

For Sensitive Skin. Homemade herbal soaps have no strong chemicals that are harsh to the skin thus they can be used for sensitive skin leaving your skin smooth and supple. They can even be used for babies because they do not contain harsh chemicals.

Anti-bacterial. By adding essential oils such as tea tree or jojoba, your herbal soap can have anti-bacterial properties.

Moisturizing. By using olive oil or sweet almond oil in your herbal soap, your skin will remain supple, soft and younger looking because these oils helps retain skin moisture by preventing its loss and at the same time attracting external moisture to the skin. A well moisturized skin prevents dryness or flaking and makes skin sparkling clear and younger looking.

Healing. Aloe Vera and avocado oils both have healing and soothing properties good for damaged or dry skin. They are rich in vitamins A, D and E which also provides nourishment to the skin making it soft, smooth and younger looking.

Treatment. Your herbal soaps can be used to treat psoriasis, acne or eczema. Psoriasis is a skin disease that has no known cure where skin exfoliation is faster than normal. You can make herbal soaps with tea tree oil, oatmeal or honey with olive and castor oil will sooth and help relieve skin inflammation. For acne, you can use goat's milk, tea tree oil or sulfur in your soap. A combination of jojoba oil, shea butter, almond oil, palm oil, coconut oil and avocado oil makes a good treatment for eczema. Goat's milk can also be used to treat eczema. You can research on the properties of these essential oils and combine or blend them to make soaps that are specifically for the treatment of certain skin diseases or disorders.

Good for the Budget. Making your own herbal soap is a lot cheaper than commercial brands. They are made of natural plants, vegetables, fruits and seed extracts which are free of chemicals. If you really want the scent or the properties of commercial soap you can always match them with your homemade blend.

Income Generator. With the knowledge of herbal soaps and the use of essential oils you can build a business out of making herbal soaps. You can start small and slowly expand your business and at the same time you get to maintain your beautiful skin.

Herbal soaps may truly be the answer to a youthful you and the panacea to all of your skin problems. It will also help you maintain your beautiful skin without the need to spend so much money on creams and lotions, dermatologists or skin clinics.

Herbal soap making consists of natural ingredients, juice, extracts and vitamins all coming from fresh medicinal plants. The intricacy of mixing different herbs makes the job enjoyable and challenging. With artistry and creative imagination it is surprisingly fun to come up with one's own unique combination.

Aside from the fancy and amazing feeling you get from this venture today, herbal or anything natural is much appreciated and sought after. Furthermore, making it right at the four corners of your home makes it more magnificent.

Herbs are natural and are safe but those with sensitive skin should also be vigilant of herbs that may irritate the skin. How to make herbal soaps are generally the same as with the other soap making only the trickiest part of it is choosing the appropriate herbs for the family.

Consider using mint for everyday soaps to enhance that invigorating effect and add it with a soothing fragrance of lavender. To achieve that whitening effect that most men and women desire is to use herbs such as kalamansi, kamias or papaya.

On the other hand avocado and cucumber are best for beauty soap. To draw forth medicinal benefits, use akapulco or guava. They have an anti-fungal or antiseptic composition. Blending and combining different herbs may also be experimented and provides the opportunity to come up with a new and unique herbal soap.

The first thing you should do is to prepare the utensils needed when making the soap. As a beginner, the tools needed might be just around the kitchen, so check it first. Buy what is lacking in the nearest store where you live. Make sure to have the following basic ingredient which is your base soap. It can be glycerin, ivory or any other unscented mild soap.

Have these following items ready as well: plastic pail, wooden ladle, glass or cup, mortar and pestle, cheese cloth or strainer, knife, chopping board, cooking pot which is preferably made of enamel, clay, stainless or glass and of course the molders. The most important of all is the stove where you will do the cooking.

Once you have all these equipments and have decided which herb to use, there are no more obstacles to keep you from starting your own herbal soap making endeavor. As a beginner start with the melt and pour method which is the easiest way to learn how to do it. Here are the step-by-step methods that are easy to follow:

1. Bring 1/4 cup of water to a boil and then add finely ground herbs that you like about 2 teaspoons and let it steep in 15 minutes.

2. Reheat the steeped concoction in a double broiler.

3. Pour in the grated or chopped based soap and melt. If coloring or fragrance oils are desired it is best to pour it in at this point of the process.

4. When the soap mix and other additives are completely melted, it is time to pour the solution in the mold. Set aside and leave in a room temperature to allow hardening for a few hours. For easy removal of soap from it's mold rub the mold first with vegetable oil before pouring the soap solution.

5. Unmold the soap after a few hours when the soap is hard enough and allow hardening process for another day or two before using it.

Keep in mind to use glass or plastic spoons and containers rather than metals since herbs may react to metals. Herbal soap making is indeed simple and easy. With just a few hours of fun and a touch of labor can provide stimulation of your body with all natural cleansing soaps

Basic Recipe Ingredients For Cold Process Herbal SoapsWhen looking through the thousands of recipes available be certain that the following ingredients are included in the basic recipe. An excellent, gentle and beneficial facial soap prepared using the cold process method would include the following ingredients:

- 5 % Castor oil

- 10% canola oil

- 10% sunflower oil

- 25% olive oil

- 25% palm oil

- 25% coconut oil

Basic Recipe Ingredients For Melt And Pour Herbal Soap Bases

- All vegetable oil. Never use any animal oil. Animal oils leave a film and soapy residue.

- No drying alcohol

- Glycerin, this is a natural moisturizer that draws moisture from the air and is extremely beneficial for dry skin

- Distilled and deodorized clear coconut oil which creates creaminess and lather.

- Shea butter bases and goats milk bases are also excellent choices for dry or sensitive skin

How to Make Natural Soap

Soap making can be very simple or you can make it as

complicated as you like.

First, the beauty of making your own is that you can make it with the ingredients that you choose and the fragrances that you like. And adjustments aren't hard but do take some practice. Further, most homemade soap recipes use ounces or grams and ingredients must be weighed to get good results. But I've found a way to simplify the process by converting the ingredients to cups and portions of cups. Consequently, it's much easier and you get the same results time after time.

Lye in Homemade Soap

The one thing in homemade soap you can't substitute is lye. You should always use 100% sodium hydroxide, or lye in crystal form. Don't substitute liquid lye or drain cleaners such as Drano. These may cause inaccurate measurements or have bits of metal in them. You don't want either.

Lye is caustic. It can eat holes in fabric and cause burns on your skin. Always be extra careful when using lye. Use gloves and eye protection and a mask if desired. When you mix the lye with water, it will heat up and fume for about 30 seconds to a minute. It may cause a choking sensation in your throat. Don't worry, it's not permanent and will go away after a few minutes. Always add lye to water (not water to lye), and start stirring right away. If allowed to clump on the bottom, it could heat up all at once and cause an explosion.

No Lye in Finished Soap

Even though lye is caustic and dangerous to work with, after it reacts with the oils in your soap (through a process called saponification), no lye will remain in the finished product.

The lye reacts with the oils, turning what starts out as a liquid into blocks of soap. When made properly, no lye remains in the finished product.

Homemade Soap Making Equipment

When learning how to make soap, remember to use equipment that will not be used for cooking. While you could clean everything really well, it's best not to take a chance.

Stainless steel, tempered glass, and enamel are all good choices for mixing bowls. Don't use copper or aluminum, they will react with the lye. Some plastics may melt, so don't use plastic bowls.

For spoons, use styrene plastic or silicone. For molds, you can get soap molds at your local craft store or online here, or use silicone baking pans (like this). These are great because you can peel the mold right off. Other things you want to have are a pint and a quart canning jar, newspaper, a stainless steel thermometer that reads between 90° and 200° (find it here), an old towel, and any additions you want to add to the soap.

How to Make Soap: The Additives

There are as many variations of soap as there are colors in the rainbow. You can literally do almost anything. Here are the basics of additives:

Herbs

All herbal material must be dried. Lavender is popular, as well as chamomile. I love lemongrass and oakmoss, though not together. Use about ¼ cup of dried plant material per batch of this size. (Find high quality dried herbs here.)

Essential Oils

Essential oils are from plants. They come from the roots, stems, flowers or seeds. Fragrance oils can be blends of essential oils or they can be artificially produced. Be sure you know what you have. Most oils can be used at the rate of 15-20 drops or around a teaspoon per batch of this size. (Find 100% pure essential oils here.)

Colors

Natural colors are easy. Use cinnamon or cocoa powder for a brown soap, powdered chlorophyll for green, turmeric for yellow and beetroot for orange. However, sometimes things change colors, like magenta beet powder turning yellowish orange. I would avoid food colors since they don't hold up well in soap. Check out our article, 44 Ways to Color Homemade Soap Naturally, for even more ideas.

Other Items

This would include aloe vera gel, oatmeal, dry milk powder, clays, cornmeal, ground coffee, salt and anything else you may want to use.

How to Make Soap for Hand & Body

Yield 5 3.5 Ounce Bars

Ingredients

- coconut oil ⅔ cup – to produce good lather (buy it in bulk here for soap making here)

- olive oil ⅔cup – which makes a hard and mild bar

- other li□uid oil ⅔ cup – like almond oil, grapeseed, sunflower or safflower oil (find them here)

- ¼ cup lye – also called 100% sodium hydroxide (find it here or at local hardware stores)

- ¾ cup cool water – use distilled or purified

Instructions

Step One

Cover your work area with newspaper. Put your gloves and other protective wear on. Measure your water into the quart canning jar. Have a spoon ready. Measure your lye, making sure you have exactly ¼ cup. Slowly pour the lye into the water, stirring as you go. Stand back while you stir to avoid the fumes. When the water starts to clear, you can allow it to sit while you move to the next step.

Step 2

In the pint jar, add your three oils together. They should just make a pint. Heat in a microwave for about a minute, or place the jar of oils in a pan of water to heat. Check the temperature of your oils – it should be about 120° or so. Your lye should have come down by then to about 120°. Wait for both to cool somewhere between 95° and 105°. This is critical for soap making. Too low and it'll come together quickly, but be coarse and crumbly.

Step 3

When both the lye and oils are at the right temperature, pour the oils into a mixing bowl. Slowly add the lye, stirring until it's all mixed. Stir by hand for a full 5 minutes. It's very important to get as much of the lye in contact with as much of the soap as possible. After about 5 minutes, you can keep stirring or you can use an immersion blender (like this). The soap mixture will lighten in color and become thick. When it looks like vanilla pudding it's at "trace" and you're good to go. (Watch this video to see what trace looks like.)

Step 4

Add your herbs, essential oils or other additions at this point. Stir thoroughly to combine. Pour the mixture into mold(s) and cover with plastic wrap. Set in an old towel and wrap it up. This will keep the residual heat in and start the saponification process. Saponification is the process of the base ingredients becoming soap.

Step 5

After 24 hours, check your soap. If it's still warm or soft, allow it to sit another 12-24 hours. When it's cold and firm, turn it out onto a piece of parchment paper or baking rack. If using a loaf pan as your mold, cut into bars at this point. Allow soap to cure for 4 weeks or so. Be sure to turn it over once a week to expose all the sides to air (which is not necessary if using a baking rack). For a DIY soap drying rack, I took an old potato chip rack and slid cardboard fabric bolts (from a fabric store) through the rungs.

Step 6

When your soap is fully cured, wrap it in wax paper or keep it in an airtight container. Hand made soap creates its own glycerin, which is a humectant, pulling moisture from the air. It should be wrapped to keep it from attracting dust and debris with the moisture.

(Notes)

When you're done making soap, always clean your equipment that has been exposed to lye. You can neutralize the lye with white vinegar, then wash the equipment well as you normally would. For the rest of it, let it sit for several days. Why? Because when you first make soap, it's all fat and lye. You'll be washing forever and you could burn your hands on the residual lye. If you wait, it becomes soap and all it takes to clean it is a soak in hot water.

Herbalism

Herbalism is my secret passion. I find all the dynamics and intricacies of each plant to be fascinating. After all, herbs have been used medicinally and for pure enjoyment for thousands of years. I, therefore, love using herbs in my homemade soapmaking. Whether you are a die hard cold-process soapmaker, hot-processor, or just like to do a little melt and pour for fun every now and then, you can include herbs in your soapmaking projects for medicinal purposes, color, exfoliation, or as a decoration to the top.

Yarrow

Yarrow While yarrow is often used internally, it is also used topically to fight against inflammation and help heal wounds faster due to its antibacterial and antiseptic properties. This makes it great for acne, eczema, and other skin conditions. Yarrow has tiny white flowers that can be dried and used on top or within soap. Leaves and flowers can be used in an herbal oil infusion and/or tea for the lye water in your soap recipe. It grows throughout North America, so you may find something blooming June through October.

Chamomile

Chamomile has traditionally been used for its calming effect in teas. It is also used topically on scars and wounds as an antibacterial, anti-inflammatory herb that is high in antioxidants. The flowers are very pretty on top of soaps and can give added medicinal properties in a tea infusion. I also like to use the petals mixed in soap for a pretty texture and visual appeal. It can also be infused through oil, giving your soap a slight golden color.

Peppermint

Peppermint is something that is easy to get a hold of or grow (it'll take over your yard), making it a fun herb to add to soaps. Like other herbs, make sure that you steep the leaves before use so they do not "bleed," making brown spots in your soap. Peppermint is often used as an exfoliant in soap, but paired with peppermint essential oil, it can create a very invigorating start to the morning.

Lemon Balm

Lemon balm is one of my favorite plants. It doesn't have showy flowers, but it just looks pretty. Actually, it looks a lot like mint when it is growing, but has a more uniform domed appearance. Recent studies have shown the benefits of lemon balm on cold sores due to the calming, relaxing, effect on the nervous system – making it beneficial for those wanting a calming aromatherapy soap, whether they get cold sores or not.

Calendula

Calendula is another great herb for calming the skin and reducing inflammation. It has beautiful yellow or orange petals that are very pretty within or on top of soap. Make an oil infusion for a golden effect to your soap.

Jewelweed

Jewelweed soap for poison ivy every year. It blooms by streams and on roadsides everywhere here in Pennsylvania, making it easy to identify and use. It has been shown to dissolve the urushiol oil that poison ivy or poison oak leaves on the skin, making it very valuable to those who suffer severe reactions. It's not something that you'll find in dried form online, so if it doesn't grow near you, then goldenseal is a good substitution if you're trying to make a poison ivy soap. I infuse the water and the bulk of the oil for soap.

Goldenseal

Goldenseal has pretty three to five lobed leaves with a flower and then fruit sticking seemingly right out of the middle. Because goldenseal is endangered from being over-harvested in the wild, be sure to only use cultivated goldenseal. Goldenseal salves are wonderful for wounds, rashes, itchiness, poison ivy, cold sores, and inflammation. Therefore, using it in soap just seems like common sense. It is sold commonly in capsules, but for soapmaking purposes, using loose-leaf goldenseal or a tea bag for a hot oil and water infusion is much more simple.

Nettles are high in vitamins and minerals. Its astringent and anti-inflammatory properties make it excellent for skin and hair. Nettle is anti-inflammatory and is calming for your skin, making it great for acne!

It can be infused in oil to give a pretty green color to your soap. The more you use, the darker green it will be.

Lavender

Lavender has always been a very popular herb to use in soapmaking. It will most likely brown when added inside the soap, which is why I like to use it on top where the small, elongated purple flowers make a beautiful addition.

Cornflowers

Cornflowers, or bachelor's buttons, are very pretty little flowers with a bright purplish blue color. Traditionally they have been used as teas to help eyesight. They are often used today to strengthen maturing skin due to their high antioxidant properties. They will turn a yellow color instead of brown if stirred into the soap, so don't be afraid to use them that way and leave some sprinkled on the top to retain that beautiful blue spark of color. While there are so many more herbs to use within soaps (rose petals, comfrey leaf, rosemary, etc.), those are my favorite

CHAPTER SEVEN

SOAP MAKING RECIPE FOR THE HOLIDAYS

Christmas is just around the corner! Have you found the perfect Christmas gifts yet? Why not make your own gift with elegant soaps the they will love and cherish.

With simple soap making recipe you can easily create elegant soaps

Here is a simple soap making recipe for those of you who haven't tried making soap yet.

A lovely gift idea for friends and family would be to make your own homemade soap. A personalized gift that you made yourself would proclaim so much more thoughtfulness than just buying one.

Making olive oil soap is fairly simple and easy.

Homemade olive oil recipe

Soap making ingredients:

One 18 ounce can of lye (Make sure the lye is labeled for soap making. Some lye are too harsh, while some others are not strong enough to make soap with)

Distilled water-5 cups (plain tap water has chemicals

and impurities that can cause soap making problems)

- Heat proof container for mixing the lye

- Large stainless steel pot for mixing soap

- Spatula (rubber or silicon)

- Plastic container with lid (which will serve as the soap making mold)

- Blender or beater

How to make the soap:

- Before starting, make sure to read carefully the Manufacturer Safety Data Sheet on the lye. Lye must be handled with extreme caution.

Please always note that when you are using Lye that Safety is top priority.

- Pour the distilled water into the heat proof container. Then add lye carefully.

Always remember:

Add lye to the water and not the other way around.

Stir gently and with care. The mixture will get hot and will produce fumes for a few minutes.

Set the mixture aside to a safe place and wait for it to cool off.

- Pour olive oil into the other large stainless

steel pot and heat to approximately 100 degrees Fahrenheit.

Then remove the pot from the heat.

- Once the container of the lye-water mixture is warm enough to touch, slowly pour the lye-water mixture into the warm olive oil, stirring the oil the whole time with your spatula.

Then, you can now use your stick bender or beater for short intervals, hand stirring in between.

You will notice the mixture starts getting thicker and more opaque which means trace is occurring.

Keep stirring until you see a pudding-like consistency.

- Pour mixture into the plastic container with lid and cover with a blanket.

When it's ready, pop it out from the container and stack it on brown paper lined shelves in a well ventilated area.

It takes approximately 4 weeks for soap to be aged and cured.

This recipe makes more than 10 pounds of soap.

Pack it any way you want it for a more personalized touch. Let your creativity run wild and don't be afraid to use color and creative materials.

These handmade soaps will now be perfect Holiday gifts for your friends and family!

Reasons to Make Handmade Soap

Are you toying with the idea of soap making as a new hobby? Not only is it fun but it's also a very practical hobby. Here are 5 reasons that will help you solidify your decision so you can stop thinking about it and start doing it.

Handmade Soap makes a Perfect Gift

Handmade soaps are the perfect gift to give for all occasions, showers, weddings, birthdays, and holidays. Rather than buying an expensive gift that will be used once or twice then sold in a garage sale, a gift of your own soap shows that you truly care about someone's health and well being. As an added benefit, homemade organic soap is inexpensive and easy to make.

You Control the Scent

If you have used store bought soap with lavender fragrance, and then used a homemade version, you will know there is a huge difference in the aroma. After bathing, the delicate perfume should linger, recalling the lush countryside of Provence. What if the traditional soap smells of citrus, rose, lavender, or vanilla are not what you are looking for in your soap?

By making handmade soaps, you can add your favorite scents to your soaps. Woody notes, such as sandalwood or patchouli, spice notes like coriander and cinnamon and leather notes of musk, moss and ambergris. Do you have a favorite perfume? Try recreating its scent by using a wide variety of essential oils.

Allergen Reduction

Store bought, mass produced soaps are usually hard soaps that dry your skin and promote flaking. The harsh chemicals can react with your skin, making it itchy and red. Many people are allergic to store bought soap and they do not even realize it! By contrast, making handmade soaps lets you control what is in your soap. Because you make it in small quantities, you can make the soft, wonderful soaps people will remember and love. Handmade soap is all-natural, made with higher quantities of fat and natural moisturizers.

You Control the Size, Shape and Color

It's your soap. You control the size and shape of your soap. Do you want tiny decorative bath soaps that resemble flowers? You can make them. Do you want a rustic looking brick of fragrant soap with no designs at all? You can make that too. As you become more proficient in the soap maker's art, you will be able to make soaps that have veins of colored clay running through them like marble and delicate translucent soaps with ripples and folds resembling antique glass. You can add natural exfoliates to your soaps as well, such as poppy seeds, coffee grounds, ground loofah, and ground oatmeal.

Your Personal Masterworks

Making handmade soaps can be a rewarding process. As you develop skill and authority in this ancient art, you may find customers that want you to make them personal soaps. Like the rich and famous, everyone enjoys having an exclusive item. You may find your soap is the best kept secret of someone's family. Best of all, soap is always something you need more of, so you can create new masterworks every time you make soap.

Types of Soap Making Molds You Can Work With

Being a newbie in soap making and to be able to appreciate your homemade soaps, you would have to pour them into your soap making molds for them to take in their final shape. This is where the fun of soap making begins! You may want to make your own molds or buy them off-the-shelf at your local craft supplies store but whichever you decide to do you still need to know what types of soap making molds you can choose from. In terms of shape and size, the following types are available:

Standard Bar Soap Mold

The standard bar soap mold is rectangular in shape with squared or sometimes rounded edges. This type of mold is usually used to make bar soaps for daily use. The resulting soap should be easy to handle and not too small.

Innovative Log Soap Molds

The log soap mold, also known as slab mold, is innovative and convenient. It allows the user to pour in several batches of soap in the same mold. It is most convenient if you need to produce a lot of soap and it is easy to cut the soap to the desired size.

Unique Novelty Molds

Novelty molds come in unique and varied shapes and sizes. There are a lot to choose from ranging from basic shapes like flowers, hearts and butterflies to fun shapes like bears, frogs and crayons to intricate designs for special occasions like Christmas, Halloween or Thanksgiving.

Customized Molds

If you have your own idea or design for your

handmade soaps then you can have your design custom-made or made just for you. This is usually done if you have your own logo for your business or company.

In choosing your molds you should also base your choice on the type of soap process you use to make your soaps. You can choose from several types of mold materials like:

Basic Soap Molds

The least expensive type of mold because it is made of plastic. However, the use of this kind of mold is best suited for cold processed soaps. It can be used for melt and pour processed soaps if the plastic mold is microwave safe.

Wooden Soap Molds

This traditional type of mold material is in the shape of a box and made of wood. It is usually designed with hinges on two sides so that the user will just need to open the box to take out the hardened soap. Before pouring in the soap mixture, you will have to put a wax paper lining so that the soap will not stick to the wood.

Silicone Soap Molds

The latest and newest fad in the soap making industry

is the use of silicone soap molds. These molds are very popular because they are very durable, flexible, non-stick and heat resistant. Customized molds are usually made of silicone.

In reality, you can make your own soap mold if you are that creative. A lot of materials are available at home which you can use. It will just need lots of your imagination to be able to use them.

Soap Making Mold - Let Your Imagination Run Wild!

In making bar soaps, using a soap making mold is quite necessary. You cannot complete your soap making process without pouring your liquid soap into a mold. And since it is an essential part of your process of making soap, why not make this step a very exciting one to highlight your experience.

There are countless molds to choose from. There are those which are readily available in crafts stores or even hardware stores. But there are soap making mold that can also be found inside your house. Yes, you read me right...in your own house. Practically anything that can hold a liquid mixture can be a soap mold. You just have to be creative in looking at things. Take for instance a wooden salad spoon. The deeper the spoon, the better it is.

I can attest to the flexibility of this famous kitchen

utensil because I used it once as a soap making mold. I was in a rush to attend a simple all-girls night out with former high school classmates. And I wanted to use this opportunity to give out samples of my homemade soap. I was just starting with my business and I want to get as many prospects as possible. So I thought why not use the occasion to my advantage.

But I don't have a readily available mold and I can't leave the house to buy. So a sparkling idea came to mind. Why not use what is within my reach? And the first thing I saw, since I was in the kitchen preparing dinner, is my salad spoon. The shape is oval and the material is perfect because then if I will only put a parchment paper before pouring the soap mixture, I can easily take out the molded soap.

I also tried using a plastic cup. The shape can be unexciting but I put some hand painted decoration to put some character into the soap. I also saw a heart-shaped silicone container. I am not sure for what purpose is this, but I saw it kept somewhere so I thought that perhaps it can also be used as a soap making mold. And viola! The soap turned out to be a great gift.

When it comes to making soap, you can let your imagination run wild. And one easy way to do this is to be creative with the choice of soap making mold to use. You can even make a thematic set of soap for any occasion. It can be a great party give-away. Weddings, birthdays, christening, anniversaries, corporate events...the occasion is boundless. And if you are seriously into the soap making business, you can make your thematic soaps using various types of molds in advanced. And you can just keep them for future orders. Just remember to secure them tight so you don't lose the quality of your homemade soap.

Organic Soap Making Supplies and Materials

In any soap making activity like organic soap making, the first thing you need to know before you start making your soap is what supplies or ingredients you need to have on hand. The supplies you will need to prepare will depend on the type of soap you are going to make. For making organic soap, you will need to prepare the following supplies:

Soap Base. A soap base makes soap making fast and easy. It is very handy and is usually used in the melt and pour process of soap making. Just like raw soap, a soap base contains essential oils, oil fragrances and colorants. Soap bases come in different varieties such as glycerine, castile, goat milk, shea butter, cocoa butter and specialty bases like olive oil, honey and oatmeal. Soap bases also come in two forms: soap base bars and shredded soap base.

Lye. Lye is also known as Caustic Soda. It is used in cold process soap making where water and lard or fats are added to it. Lye comes in solid dry form such as flakes, pellets, powder, beads and in solution form and dissolved in water. Lye is a corrosive chemical and can cause burns and injury to the skin and blindness if it reaches the eyes.

Carrier Oil. Carrier oil is also known as vegetable oil or base oil. It is used to dilute the essential oils and help these oils to get into the skin. Most carrier oils come from pressed vegetables, fruit seeds or nuts such as olive oil, grape seed oil, sunflower seed, avocado, canola (rapeseed), sesame, jojoba, sweet almond, pecan, walnut and macadamia.

Essential Oils or Fragrance. Essential oils are also known as volatile or ethereal oils. They are extracted from plants and are extracted for their aroma or fragrance. They are used in combination with carrier oils to add fragrance to your organic soaps. Essential oils are extracted from various parts of plants:

1. Seeds - almond, anise, cumin, nutmeg

2. Flowers   -   lavender,   rose,   ylang-ylang, chamomile, sage, geranium

3. Leaves - basil, cinnamon, eucalyptus, lemon grass, peppermint

4. Peel - orange, lemon, lime, grapefruit

5. Wood - cedar, sandalwood, camphor

Natural Ingredients. Natural ingredients are extracts or ingredients added to a soap base mixture to give the soap a unique and distinctive characteristic. There are several varieties of natural ingredients that can be used in soaps for different purposes as:

1. Exfoliants - oatmeal, poppy seeds, sugar, salt, corn meal

2. Cleansing - grapefruit seed extract, milk

3. Relaxant - honey, lavender, rosemary

4. Moisturizer - shea butter, wheat germ, aloe vera, cocoa butter

Molds. Molds are the containers wherein the soap mixture is poured on and left to harden and take shape. Soap molds come in a variety of shapes, sizes and materials. There are also novelty soaps for special occasions and you can have molds customized for specific needs.

Colorants. Colorants are used to give color to your soap. Food coloring can be used as colorant. Pigments and micas come in different colors. There are also earth tone metallic micas and glitters that can make add intensity to your soap and make it visually attractive.

Equipments. Equipments such as stainless steel pots or pans, double boiler pans, mixing bowls, miller or blender, and a stove or microwave are some of the equipments you will need in making your organic soap.

Utensils and safety equipments. You will also need goggles and rubber gloves for safely handling the hazardous substances such as lye. A weighing scale to measure your ingredients, plastic or stainless steel spoons for mixing, thermometer, pitcher, aprons and pot holders.

The above enumerated supplies are also basic requirements for making natural, herbal soaps and other kinds of soap.

Synthetic Soap - Coloring Option

Many soap-makers prefer to use natural soap making colorants for their soaps, as opposed to synthetic ones. However, if the natural colorants don't work for you, or are too expensive or unpredictable, there are a variety of synthetic colorants that can be used.

Pigments, micas, and FD&C colorants are some of these.

Pigments are colorants that were originally mined, but now, due to FDA regulations, are manufactured in laboratories.

Many natural oxides contain toxic materials, so the

FDA chose to approve only synthetic colorants for use in soaps and cosmetics.

The synthetically made pigments have the same molecular structure as the natural ones, but they have a low enough concentration of toxic metals that they are considered "safe" by the FDA. Pigments tend to be pretty stable, and the color that they will impart to your soap is predictable. The liquids are extremely easy to use, but the powders must be mixed with liquid before they are added to the soap batter, and they may clump.

The easiest way to liquefy the colorant powder is to:

Put a tiny bit of rubbing alcohol into a bowl - ¼ teaspoon is probably enough - and then add some powder.

Mix until all of the powder has dissolved in the alcohol. Mix the solution into the soap batter at the correct stage; if the batter is not your desired hue, mix more colorant solution. Another method of mixing the powdered colorant is to combine it with liquid glycerin, in a ratio of 2 parts glycerin to 1 part colorant powder. (The advantage of the liquid colorants is that this process is unnecessary; the colorant can be added, one drop at a time, until the soap has achieved the desired hue.)

FD&C colorants are also manufactured in a laboratory. By way of comparison, they are easier to use than many pigments, and provide a much wider range of colors. There is some debate over the safety of FD&C colorants, because in the past, the FDA has recalled some of these colorants due to safety concerns. However, this fear is, most likely, unfounded.

FD&C colorants are in almost all of the processed foods we eat, so the miniscule amount that is in soap is not really cause for concern.

FD&C colorants are inexpensive, and very easy to use; they are great for use in melt-and-pour soap, but they don't usually remain stable in cold-process soap, due to its high alkalinity.

Micas are a combination of natural and synthetic materials. The micas themselves are natural material; after they are mined, they are then coated with FD&C colorants, or pigments, to provide them with color. Shimmery micas are normally used to give color to makeup, but can be used for soap as well. Because of their metallic sheen, micas can only display their color by reflecting light; therefore, they work best in translucent soaps. They blend very smoothly, but a larger amount is required than if you were coloring the soap with other colorants.

Micas also look nice in cold-process soap, but because

some of them are coated with FD&C colorants, they should be tested before use.

When the colorant you used transfers unintentionally, and alters the look of the intended design, this is referred to as bleeding, or color migration. This usually occurs in melt-and-pour soaps, because water is mixed with the soap base to melt it, and many colorants are water-soluble.

Therefore, if you want to make a soap that, instead of being a solid color, has a pattern or design, your best bet is to use colorants that are oil-soluble; another option is to use colorants that aren't soluble, and color the soap via dispersion (meaning that the particles are suspended throughout the soap, instead of being dissolved in it). Oxides and most micas will color soap without bleeding.

Liquid Soap

Liquid soap is the most efficient cost cutter for businesses and home consumers, and a product that is popular with users. There is less waste with soap products than you experience with other hard soaps, and there is better germ control with less mess when you provide soap at home or in the business setting. Popular brand name liquid hand soaps are Gojo, Dial and Softsoap. These are major brand names that everyone knows and enjoys using.

When you purchase liquid hand soap online, you get many advantages including a wide choice of soap products, fast delivery service, and the ability to shop for wholesale pricing. Typically, online stores deliver anywhere in the continental United States from warehouses nearest your location.

Using liquid soap is the preference for businesses, due to cost efficiency. Soap dispensers give each user the proper amount of soap, so there is less waste and better use of soap inventories. Cleaning the sink areas is much easier, as the soap is quickly cleaned up with no residue. There are no messy soapy bars that leave scum and germs behind when you provide liquid soap. This also makes using soap preferable for home use. Liquid soap is easier for children to use, again with less mess and less waste of product.

Gojo, Dial and Softsoap are well known brand name soaps that people trust. They have a light fragrance or can be purchased fragrance free, and create a nice cleaning lather with just a small amount of water. You can purchase these brands, dispensers, and paper products at discount pricing. Most online janitorial stores supply home consumers and businesses across the country with fast delivery and excellent customer service year round.

Liquid soap is just as important for home use as it is in the business world. Liquid soaps are available in many variations and containers that are suitable for home use. Attractive dispensers fit right into home décor and business settings, and there is no need for a messy bar soap dish. Home consumers can get the same wholesale discount pricing that larger businesses enjoy by shopping online.

Selecting the best type of liquid hand soap product for your home or business is easy online. Soaps are the number one choice for hospitals, doctor's offices, nursing homes, and schools. Liquid soap is also recommended by the CDC to help stop the spread of germs causing illnesses and infections. Hand washing is the best prevention against catching germs before consuming food or touching your face. Using soap makes this process of hand washing easier. Be sure to browse our janitorial supply web sites for a wide selection of "Liquid Soap" and other cleaning supplies and janitorial products!

Aromatherapy Soaps

As with any kind of aromatherapy, aromatherapy soaps are going to help relax you while rejuvenating your overall body in the bathtub or shower. These soaps contain therapeutic aromatherapy oils from natural herbs and plants. There are a number of different kinds of natural soap to choose from and each is made from a different kind of essential oil.

Something few people link with aromatherapy is skin treatment. One of the biggest causes of dry skin that breaks out is the use of harsh soap. This all natural soap is made from ingredients that are gentle to the skin, thus helping reduce the effects of acne.

As you shop for these kinds of soaps, it is vital you only purchase kinds with all natural ingredients. Pure and natural soap is going to give you the best results for whatever it is you are looking for. There are a number of soaps that contain other ingredients as well that simply will not give you the same results.

If you are a crafty person and are interested, handmade natural soap is an option. You can use this handmade soap for yourself, as a gift, or sell them to friends and family. The important thing to remember if you are going to make your own handmade natural soap is that you use all natural ingredients. Make sure to purchase quality ingredients that are 100 percent natural.

If you purchase poor quality ingredients, your soap is going to break and crack fairly quickly. You can purchase soap molds and ingredients at craft stores or on the internet. You can even find aromatherapy soap starter kits to help you get going.

There are several different kinds of body and bath aromatherapy soaps to look for. Some of the more popular kinds include rose, chamomile and ylang ylang oil as each of these has a romantic essence. This provides a great deal of relaxation to relieve yourself of any stresses and worries.

There are a number of different benefits to using aromatherapy soaps over other kinds of essential oils. Typically, essential oils are going to be used solely in a bathtub. However, having soaps gives you the ability to take advantage of natural soap in the shower as well. In addition, you can apply the soap to specific areas that are sore or achy.

The number one thing you want to look for with aromatherapy soaps is 100 percent all natural soap ingredients. If you purchase anything different, you are not going to get the full effects.

Common Mistakes in the Soap Making Process

Your first soap making process does not always give you the results you are looking for. A ruined batch of soap also means a loss of time, money and most of all, the ingredients. Doing a test before you proceed with your soap making is very helpful. Just like any activity, natural soap making is a trial and error method.

Below is a list of some common mistakes in the soap making process.

Making a huge batch of soap.

In business, the motto is start small, think big. This

also holds true for your soap making process. There is always a chance that the recipe you have never used before can create problems with your batch of soap. Therefore if you make a huge batch, many of those ingredients will be wasted. Try using two pounds as a safe test size. If it works, then there is a higher chance that your larger batch will come out perfect.

Changing multiple ingredients.

Experimenting with ingredients in the soap making process is good as you progress in the activity. However at the start, it is preferable for you to use a recipe that has been tried and tested. Refrain from changing more than one ingredient at a time in a recipe if you do not know what each ingredient will add or take away from the soap.

Putting in too many additional ingredients.

Soap making is indeed a fun activity and as you become familiar with the process, you cannot help but try experimenting with the ingredients. You are free to add whatever fragrance you choose; additives such as olive oil, essential oils, sodium hydroxide and coloring. However, sometimes, adding too many ingredients can become a disaster, as it can completely ruin your soap. For example, if you use too much fragrance in your soap, the fragrance will thin out the product and it will be impossible to repair the damage.

Lack of patience.

The soap making process does not end within an hour after your soaps are done. Soap is best when you allow ample time for the formulations to sit. Natural ingredients could take a few months if they are not combined at the right temperature. You can label your soap by batches and number and check every now and then to make sure that they are still stable. Note how long the fragrance lasts and check to see if your soap shrinks from the wrapper.

Not writing down soap making instructions.

The more you make soap, the basics will start to become very simple and you can do it automatically. However do not think that you can remember everything, especially when you start making many different kinds of soaps. Write it down and keep a journal that you can check out every now and then. You may even wish to separate your work into different categories such as liquid soap, or solid, whether you used a hot process and even compile lists of your soap supplies. After all, soap making is not the only activity you do around the house. This way, you will have a fantastic resource, that you can refer to anytime you need it.

Putting in fragrance without testing.

You often make changes in your soap recipe and

mostly on the fragrance. Fragrance oils are just one aspect of the basic elements of your soap and experimenting with them can be a lot of fun. However if you are not sure about what the fragrance can do to your soap, it is best to test it first. Test the fragrance oil in a small batch of soap before you decide to add it to your larger batch. Essential oils are expensive yet provide a beautiful scent to your natural soap, so be careful and do not forget to keep instructions for yourself. Soon you will have some great soaps that will not only smell terrific but provide effective skin care too.

Making Heavenly Vanilla Soap Using The Melt and Pour Process

Have you ever been to a beauty shop and smelled the aroma of absolutely gorgeous hand-made soap and thought to yourself, "I wish I could do something like this"? Well, the good news is that you can, with the right tools, know-how and imagination.

So why should you make your own soap? Not only is it fun and exciting, but you get to put exactly what you want in it, design it how you like and choose the colors and fragrance as well. Some store-bought soaps can be full of chemicals that can be harmful to the skin, but if you make your own you know exactly what is in it.

What is the melt and pour process? The melt and

pour process is exactly how it sounds. You use ready-made blocks of soap that are uncolored and unscented and you melt the soap blocks. Then you add your own colors, fragrances and/or other additives, pour it in a mold and wait until it's set. Melt and pour soap bases are available from online soap suppliers or craft stores. One of the advantages of using the melt and pour process to make soap is that you don't have to deal with potentially dangerous lye.

The equipment you will need will depend entirely on the soap that you are creating. You'll need either a double boiler or sturdy heat resistant microwave bowl or jug to melt the soap in and a base or mold for the shape of the soap. Also, a couple of whisks or spoons and a set of measuring spoons for additives. These are the basic tools you'll need and then you can add absolutely anything you want from there on.

Before you start, it is good to bear in mind that the soap can be extremely hot when it has been melted, so it is best to be very careful. If you're using the microwave, make sure you wear protective gloves and use a sturdy potholder to take out the microwave bowl or jug containing the hot melted soap. It's also a good idea to wear gloves if you're melting it in a double boiler, in case you accidentally splash. And make sure you're not disturbed by children or pets.

Now let's try out a basic melt and pour soap recipe called Heavenly Vanilla.

In order to make this you're going to need the following equipment:

- Clean cutting board
- Double boiler or sturdy heat resistant microwave bowl or jug, eg Pyrex
- Scales (to measure soap)
- 4 oz or 113 grams of good quality white melt and pour soap base
- Vanilla fragrance suitable for soap making
- Clean metal whisk or spoon
- Clean measuring spoons
- Clean 3-4 oz basic soap mold
- Rubbing alcohol in spray bottle
- Protective gloves
- Safety goggles
- Protective clothes
- Protective shoes

Now you have everything you need, so let's move on to the exciting part, making your own soap!

After you've put on the safety goggles, protective gloves, clothes and shoes, you can first measure the fragrance and set it aside. Start off using 0.25 ounce of fragrance per pound of soap; you can make it stronger or weaker from there. So for this recipe you would use 1.9 ml or 0.06 oz or 1/4 +1/8 US teaspoons of fragrance.

Next, weigh the soap base and melt 4 oz in either a double boiler or in the microwave. If melting it in the microwave, cover the container with Saran wrap to stop the soap from drying out. Melt the soap in one minute increments in the microwave. Stir after every minute while being careful of the hot soap base.

Once it's totally melted, it's time to add the vanilla fragrance that you've already measured and set aside. Add it slowly and stir carefully and gently. If you get bubbles at this stage it means you've stirred it too hard.

Now you're ready to pour it into the mold. Pour it very slowly and gently. Avoid splashing. If you get bubbles pouring it into the mold, spritz the surface of the soap in the mold lightly with rubbing alcohol.

Now put the mold in a safe place and leave it for a few hours. If you're in a hurry, you can put it in the refrigerator (not the freezer) for about an hour until it's set.

Once the soap is set (hardened), it's time to unmold it. Unmolding soap is just like unmolding a cake from a cake tin. Gently tap the mold then see if the soap pops out. If it doesn't it may need a further tap. If the soap is really stubborn, trying running some warm water over the bottom of the mold.

You can now use your Heavenly Vanilla soap right away!

Making soap can be good fun and the satisfaction that comes afterwards is great. So why not make your own soap today?

The Role of Glycerine in the Production of Soap

Glycerin, also spelled glycerine, is a basic ingredient in most soap. In fact, it is a by-product of soap manufacture as it occurs due to the reaction of strong alkali with an animal fat. This process is known as saponification and it is this process that brings out soap or detergent. While most manufacturers separate glycerin from the mixture, others incorporate the compound for its natural benefits.

Lots of soap-makers recommend glycerin as a basic ingredient because it has the ability to draw in moisture preventing drying of the skin. The compound is a natural moisturizer. In fact, it is a humectant - a substance that attracts water. Thus, soap containing the hygroscopic compound is known to have skin conditioning and moisturizing effect.

Glycerin is a viscous liquid that is at the same time sweet and colorless. It solidifies to a paste-like substance and has a high boiling point. During the soap-making process, some manufacturers remove the compound from the soap mixture and incorporate it into other products like lotion and creams. However, when it is added to a bar of soap it results to a nearly transparent product with moisturizing properties.

The compound is known to be a good solvent and this is one of its most remarkable properties. In some instances, it is better as a solvent than water or alcohol. This property makes it highly miscible in both alcohol and water. However, it never dissolves in oils. In its pure form the compound is called glycerol which suggests it belongs to a classification of organic compounds called alcohol.

It is extremely hygroscopic, which means that it readily absorbs moisture from the air. For instance, leaving a flask of pure glycerol open allows attraction of water that it soon loses the purity.

It was in 1889 when the compound was first obtained from animal fat through candle making. During which time the only way to derive the compound is through this process. Also, in that time animal fat was the only raw material for making candles. During the World War II, it has become a major component of dynamites and heavy demand for the substance was not sufficed by soap making industry. Thus there was an abrupt production of synthetic forms of the compound.

The substance has a chemical formula $C_3H_8O_3$ which is also occurs as a liquid by-product during the production of biodiesel in a process called transesterification. This syrupy liquid occurs in nature. Found in cells of plants and animals (including humans), it is a part of the large bio-molecules of many lipids. In biologic processes the compound occurs as a result of the fermentation of carbohydrates. In organic chemistry it is produced by propylene synthesis.

Glycerin is an ingredient in several health-care products and toiletries. It is found in food products, as well as pharmaceutical and cosmetic items. It is found in moisturizing lotions and creams because of its hydrophilic and hygroscopic properties, which allow the substance to retain moisture. There is a debate whether it is the hygroscopic properties of the compound that makes it good for the skin, or it may be possible that the chemical has other unexplored and unidentified properties aside from the one already mentioned. The moisture-drawing property makes it an excellent emollient when added in soaps and moisturizing creams. An emollient is a substance that smoothens and softens skin. Another reason personal care products utilizes the substance is because of its skin lubricating advantage, not to mention it serves as a thickening or emulsifying agent in cosmetic products.

Home-made soaps or the hand-made varieties

naturally contain glycerol, which commercial soap-makers remove. The separated liquid is used in massage oils, lip balms, skin softeners and moisturizers, perfumes and essential oils, and pharmaceutical preparations.

The Benefits of Organic Soaps Without Toxicity

When it comes to making organic soap, the idea that it will not have toxic ingredients in it is a given. If you're going to the trouble of making soap, it should be organic. It just makes sense that if you wanted various other ingredients in your soap, you could just buy it from your local store. I think in today's society, the common thinking is, the fewer the chemicals the better. I'm not so sure that we are even aware of all the benefits of using organic soaps. I think that over time these benefits will slowly make themselves known to us. We will be pleasantly surprised. I know one of the benefits of making your own soap that would be quite obvious to anyone who has purchased their own organic soap recently, and that is the high price. Store bought soaps are very expensive.

Obviously, the big advantage of making your own is the fact that you know exactly whats in it. This is so very important to the family member who suffers from allergy's. Its anybody's guess whats in some of the manufactured soaps. People today are trying to connect with their roots and getting back to basics. Many of us started out as people who's lives were quite simple and probably more focused. As time marched on those lives became more and more complicated, busy and routine. Today we are wondering what happened to those slower, simpler times. If this is starting to sound like a Norman Rockwell Painting. that's exactly what I'm going for.

My point is that so few things are natural anymore. It seems like everything we buy today is absolutely loaded with chemicals, Do you ever wonder how many of those are really necessary and how many are just there? Maybe the simple act of making organic soap is where it all starts, as far as getting back at least some of those simpler times. I think when you tie yourself to the organic movement, we will all reap what is sewn.

Remember, all fruits and vegetables cannot be touched by chemicals to call themselves a true organic. One of the more popular questions is, can I make organic soap without Lye? The answer is yes. One method is the melt and dump technique. This may involve the use of goats milk or glycerin. Make sure you put your own personal touch in your Soap, by way of shapes or fragrances. Make it a memorable experience. Well that's about it Guys. Remember, if you do this right you will definitely be glad you did.

Hand Made Soaps - Advantages and Materials

Hand made soaps, like all form of soap, are created through the process of saponification. In this, a metallic alkali reacts with fat or oil to form soap. Most soaps today are created with fats such as olive oil. Lye is used as the metallic base.

Other names for lye are sodium hydroxide and caustic soda. It is used as a strong chemical base in the industrial manufacture of many other things. These include pulp, paper, textiles, and detergents. It is also used as a drain cleaner and in the creation of drinking water.

Historically, soap was created through a hot process. Most soap today is created through the cold process method.

Hand made soaps have a lot to offer over those produced through industrial processes. When it comes to making it at home, excess fats are generally used. This serves to consume the alkali. This technique is known as "superfatting."

In the process of superfatting soap, the glycerin is not removed. Glycerin, or glycerine, is the common name for glycerol. This chemical compound is a thick liquid that is both colorless and odorless. It is widely used in medicinal applications. In addition to this area and that of personal care, it is also used for and within food and beverages.

When it comes to the creation of hand made soaps, glycerin works to create a naturally moisturizing soap (as opposed to a pure detergent.)

Superfatting may also be achieved by adding less lye, rather than extra fats.

These types of soaps, with their excess of fat, are significantly more skin-friendly than those created through industrial methods. Of course, if too much fats are included, excessive greasiness may be a result.

It is easy to see why an individual may prefer these soap options rather than industrial ones. In addition to their more mild treatment of the skin, they are just of a higher quality in general. Also, many people enjoy the organic appearance of such home made creations.

A "soaper," or person who makes soap, may choose to do this for these reasons, as well as to keep traditional practices alive. Historically, a specific area within a medieval household was responsible for the creation of wax, candles, and soap. This was known as the "chandlery." A person who made or sold candles or soap was known as a chandler.

Soap may also be created by those who have an interest in chemistry or other areas of manufacture. Today, it has become more and more common for people to choose to create organic soaps instead of utilizing synthetic detergents due to environmental concerns.

The Truth Surrounding Homemade Soap Recipes Finally Revealed

Here is an ebooks for everyone who has sat around, contemplating about the advantages of making soap from home and not spending heaps of money on it in a store or online. We will discuss the pros and cons of homemade soap, and soap recipes, as well as what it will take for you to tackle this activity. I personally have always wanted to try making soap from home, because I love doing practical activities with my free time instead of squandering it on pointless things and needing to rely on stores and outside sources for all of my home necessities. Making soap from home is not for everyone but if you take joy in doing projects especially ones that leave you with a usable, better then the store posses, product then it just might be perfect for you.

Many recent hours of my life have been devoted to learning about what homemade soap making is all about. Also why one would take this up as a pastime and what is needed to make it happen. This article is a compiled list of the best information I have gathered during my studies on soap making. Many people do not know where to look online for this type of information or do not have the time to spend hours online looking into this as I have.

There are a few different methods of making soap from home. Four of them to be precise; The Melt and Pour method; The Rebatching method; The Cold Process, and The Hot Process. Melt and Pour refers to when you purchase a pre-made block of soap, then melt it down and add fragrances; additives, and colors that you have picked out for the soap. Second is the Cold Process method, the most popular method which offers the greatest flexibility. In the Cold Process you are starting from scratch, making your own lye-solution and adding in all your own additives. This allows you to know exactly what goes into your soap and gives you the ability to truly tailor the soap to your personality and liking. The Hot Process is much the same as the Cold Process only it adds an additional step of actually cooking the soap. Rebatching is our last method and involves taking bars of soap then grinding them into a powder, adding milk or water and blending them back into bars.. Now that we know the basics of all the popular soap making methods lets take a look at my favorite one a little closer.

Once we have made the decision that we want to make soap from home and we want to use the method that gives us the most control over the ingredients in our soap, which is the Cold Process, what is the next step? We need to start by making a list of items we will need. Go ahead and grab some sturdy goggles and a nice pair of rubber gloves next time you are out, as you will need these for safety, which always comes first. We will also need large stainless pots and measuring cups. Add to that a thermometer, stick-blender, a few large wooden spoons and a mold for your soap and we are done with the hardware. Only thing left is lye and water for the lye-solution. Quick side note lye can be very dangerous and give a pretty nasty chemical burn so no messing around when using it and please wear gloves and goggles. All that is left is to gather up what you will be adding as fragrances, additives, and color for your mixture. For at least your first few batches of soap you will probably be getting these from the soap recipe you are using. It should go without saying but anything that you use for soap making should be only for soap making and labeled that way. I don't care how much you scrub I wouldn't be caught dead using any of these items for cooking food in afterwords.

I am not going to go into the step by step of how soap is made using The Cold Process, but I do want to give you a quick idea of what takes place. We begin by mixing up the lye-solution and then move on to melting the oils that our recipe calls for. We now will put these two things together and move into the adding of the rest of our ingredients, such as fragrances or colors. Stir everything together and pour into your mold and wait for it to harden. Let it cure by sitting for several weeks and you have soap. See not much to it. Of course there are more little steps then that and I do recommend finding or buying a good guide or book that will walk you through them and give you lots of tips and secrets to making your soap the best it can be.

We have equipped you with some basic tips to getting started on creating your own sweet soaps from home. You should know what you need and what you can expect. There are many great resources out there that can help and get you making soap in no-time. Before you know it you will be the master soap maker you have always dreamed of being

Starting a Soap Making Business at Home

Starting a home based soap business from your home is easy and can be quite profitable! Even a beginner can make a nice side income from making soap at home. Home based business have many advantages and a few disadvantages. The advantages are obvious, no commute, readily available for family, doing household chores while being at home, mom's taxi, etc... The disadvantages can be space, family understanding when you are 'working', getting and staying organized, etc... The rise of home based businesses is a testament that working from home can and does work everyday in the real world. Learning to balance home and business can be the best of both worlds.

The time to get started is NOW! Start producing your handcrafted soaps now so you will be ready for upcoming sales opportunities. There are endless ideas of marketing your wares, spring farmer's markets, Mother's Day, Christmas and all the other sales opportunities that crop up. Planning ahead for special occasion sales will help reduce stress when holidays and special promotions become available. Selling out at a farmers market or craft/art fair is wonderful! However, it is not wonderful if you sell out at 10 am and have paid for an entire weekend for your booth! Always look and act the part of being a professional business person. There are some crafters and artisans that plan for only a few select fairs or events per year and they truly make their money at only these affairs. Others take advantage of internet sales, local shops, and other consignment arrangements. See if there are any co-op shops in your area, co-ops are becoming increasingly popular for crafters and artisans.

Marketing and branding is the key to becoming a successful small business owner. Marketing ideas are endless! Word of mouth is a great way to get noticed on a small scale. Consider giving away your bars at first and before long friends and family will be buying from you for themselves and as gifts. Gift shops are always looking for new products to keep their stores fresh for the public. Working in cooperation with a local salon could be a great idea to get your product out there as well. Offer the salon so many free bars with a specified service of the salon. See if they will carry your new line of designer soaps even if it is for a trial basis to begin with. Baskets are always a hit at showers and you could produce specialty baskets with designer scents or themes. Again, sales ideas are endless putting those ideas in action is what will ultimately sell your product. Remember you are associated with the brand itself, you are essentially selling yourself when you sell your handcrafted soaps. Make your brand memorable in packaging and in your sales. Educate your customers about the products you produce and ingredients used. Help them in their selections and in making their own gift baskets. Creativity is the key to longevity in the small business world.

Making the soap itself, design and packaging, creating your logo are all the 'fun' parts of business. Now you must also pay attention the not so fun parts, getting sales permits, tax ID numbers and of course any and all state laws that pertain to your new enterprise. This all sounds more daunting than it is. In reality it is usually a very simple process with nothing more than filling out few forms and submitting a check. Keep accurate records of all sales and costs involved and owning your own soap making business can be a joy as well as providing extra income and when you are ready to make it a full time business! Find a good accountant for small business by asking other small business owners for referrals. You need not go to the largest accounting firm in your area, in fact I would not recommend it. The independent accountant usually works with many smaller companies and probably is a small business him/herself and understands home based businesses and what that entails.

Be willing to learn from others and join the soap making community for advice and support. Learning from the pro's can help you avoid costly mistakes. Get acquainted with all the in's and out's of soap making as a business and you too can be successful in your new endeavor!

Easy to Start, 5 Ways

A soap making business often shows up on lists of possible home-based businesses. I tried it myself and quickly was swamped with making soap and watching people haul it away.

There's more to it than first appears, but there are obvious advantages to soap making as a tiny-scale business that is easy to get going, and can be profitable, if you go about it the right way.

Not Much Cost To Start Means Low Risk

Many home business ideas look attractive and offer the chance for real profits, but the cost of entry is high, both in money and time required. Making and selling soap and related items, on the other hand, requires a very small initial investment.

The materials and equipment needed take little initial capital. You can try it out, and if you don't like what happens, you can use the product, and probably sell the little bit of equipment quite easily.

On the other hand, you probably won't fail, and you probably will make some profit.

Easy Natural Soap Production From Home

Some crafts take years to master, and much education as well, to get to the point of doing professional work. Soap making requires education and learning too, but the required time to master the basics is quite short. That means you can build a small-scale manufacturing center right at home fairly quickly.

That doesn't mean you can't continue to learn.

You can spend many years learning and improving skills, but you can also make great strides toward professional practices in short order.

They Are Ready. Are You?

That means the demand for quality handcrafted soap is there. Other have gone before you and educated many people about why handcrafted soap beats commercial soap.

The demand is there.

But many potential customers are out there looking for something new and a little different. That something new and a little different can come from you, and it's not hard to do.

Someone remarked to me not long ago that all soap is pretty much the same and it was impossible to make it unique. Wrong. It just takes a little imagination.

How Many Ways Can You Sell Soap?

Finding a new customer is the biggest challenge for any business.

You can do it many ways.

Sell through gift shops, at home parties, at craft fairs and through the mail or a catalog or even on a website. Some work better than others, and there's a good reason to start a certain way.

The Wonders Of A Soap Customer List

Once you have a customer, the easy part begins, but a typical soap maker likely doesn't know that.

See, your customers will become your friends and repeat buyers if you simply give them the chance.

That's where the easy money is, and the money you can make, while you stay at home. Follow up with customers with some easy-to-do marketing materials, and you start a real business with real value.

Starting a soap business works because it's low-risk, and easy to do. The demand for products you can produce is already there, and there are many ways to connect with people who want natural soap. They want other things too, and that's the basis for a real business if you want one. Make great soap. Find customers the easy way. Offer the ones how buy more! That's the way you do it.

Learning the Good Stuff About Soap Making

Soaps are considered a necessity in our homes. Since these are practically cleansing agents that we use, it is unlikely that a certain home will not have any of these. The use of these cleaning agents dates back during the ancient times which have been carried over to the present. Soaps are basically used for bathing, washing and cleaning. These cleansing agents are synthesized from animal or vegetable fats. When it comes to cleaning, soaps are very effective.

Soap making is just a matter or mixing the raw materials in order to make the finished products. The process of making soaps is also known as saponification. This process basically involves mixing fats and oils with a certain amount of alkali. In soap making, this mixture results in the formation of salts of fatty acids. These salts capture the dirt and grease ensuring that they will be removed from the surface. As this is washed by water, the dirt and soap mixture comes with it, leaving nothing but a clean surface.

There are different kinds of soaps which are made. Besides from the commercial ones that we are used to, there are also handmade soaps. These handmade soaps are the products that you get from making the soaps from scratch. The qualities of these two soaps are very different. In fact, making it basically involves superfatting or the addition of an excess amount of fats into the soap mixture. The main advantage of this method is to make the soap skin-friendly. As the glycerine is left untouched in the soap, it is still able to keep it moisturizing property.

There are actually different kinds of soap making processes. These are the cold process, hot process and the melt & pour process. There are certain advantages and disadvantages that these methods have. The cold process is done by slightly melting the mixture to liquefy it and maintain it at that temperature. The hot process of soap making involves heating the soap mixture to a higher temperature. For the melt & pour process, there is a pre-made mixture which is melted and poured into the mold.

Soap making is an easy process to do since the raw

ingredients needed for this is easily accessible. You can get them in your grocery stores and even in specialty craft stores. Soap making is actually a flexible activity to do. You can personalize the soaps that you make depending on your taste. It is up to you to add the color and the scent of the soaps. Whatever it is that you like, you can make it with your soaps.

Creativity makes soap making very fun! You can absolutely do anything that you want with your soaps. Don't get too excited when you make your soaps because there are certain precautionary measures that you should take. Lye is an essential ingredient in soap making, but it is very dangerous to handle. Always wear safety equipment when handling soap mixtures with lye to keep you safe all the time.

CHAPTER EIGHT

BEST HOMEMADE SOAP RECIPES:

Milk & Honey Soap

A quick DIY, this 10-minute melt and pour recipe incorporates the anti-aging, acne-fighting, clarifying, and moisturizing properties of raw organic honey with the skin soothing benefits of goat milk – no lye needed.

Tea Tree & Charcoal Facial Soap

Formulated for combination to oily skin types, this sleek and sexy black bar of soap contains the healing attributes of tea tree oil along with the detoxifying effects of activated charcoal. And the selection of skin-friendly oils like castor, coconut, palm, olive, and tamanu oils, ensures it's also deeply hydrating.

Pure Coconut Oil Soap

Requiring only four ingredients – coconut oil, water, lye, and your choice of essential oils – this basic soap is naturally moisturizing and cleansing. Using the wondrous process of "superfatting", more coconut oil is added than the lye can convert to soap, creating a bar that is extra fatty and therefore moisturizing. This recipe can also be easily adjusted to make laundry soap as well.

Aloe Vera Soap

With the ability to soothe sunburns, heal wounds, treat acne, moisturize, and defy the outward signs of aging, aloe vera is truly an amazing specimen and the perfect candidate for soapmaking. Harvest the gel from your own plant (or purchase organic aloe vera gel) and combine with coconut oil, shea butter, olive oil, lye, and lard to make this super nourishing soap.

Lavender Oatmeal Soap

A cure for dry, itching, and otherwise sensitive skin, this soap recipe combines the awesome powers of lavender with the reparative qualities of oatmeal. To make, you'll need goat's milk soap base, quick cook oats, dried lavender flowers and lavender essential oil.

Yogurt & Banana Soap

With the core ingredients of banana powder, flax seed oil, and powdered yogurt, this body bar is rife with potassium, vitamins A, E, and B6, essential fats, and lactic acid. An excellent cure for dry skin, it also contains coconut oil, castor oil, babassu oil, cocoa butter, shea butter, and olive oil.

Pink Himalayan Salt Grapefruit Soap

And in yet another way to put Himalayan salt to good use, this soap recipe calls for just three ingredients: pink Himalayan salt, goat milk soap base, and grapefruit essential oil.

Poppy Seed Soap

A poppy seed soap two ways! The lemon poppy seed version is a fantastic kitchen soap that will swiftly remove the odor of garlic and onion from the hands, while the almond poppy seed soap is akin to a lotion bar. Both are excellent exfoliants thanks to the poppy seeds.

Hemp & Shea Soap

Hemp oil is rich in omega-3 and omega-6 fatty acids, both of which are critical components for healthy skin. This soap recipe incorporates plenty of fats (shea butter, lard, coconut oil, castor oil, olive oil, and hemp seed oil) along with a goodly amount of white kaolin clay to make it extra creamy and sudsy. Top with hemp hearts for the full decorative effect.

Coffee Soap

With an intoxicating aroma, this coffee soap is a melt and pour recipe. Using a goat's milk base along with almond oil for conditioning, fresh coffee grounds for exfoliation, and your choice of fragrance (coffee cake or vanilla are both good picks), this one will surely perk you up in the morning.

Calendula Soap

Rich in antioxidants, the calendula plant has been used for centuries to heal, hydrate, and protect the skin. An excellent choice as an ingredient for homemade soap, this cold process recipe uses dried calendula petals (harvested from the plant or purchased here) infused in coconut, olive, and rice bran oil.

Soap Scrap Soap

A pennywise way to use up those bits of soap toward the end of the bar, all you need to do is save them up, chop or grate them, toss into a pot of water and set to a gentle boil. Once it's nice and hot, pour into greased molds to cool. And voila, a brand new bar of soap!

Handmade Soap Recipes

Are you looking for some easy homemade soap recipes? We've collected a ton of clever tutorials that will teach beginners how to make homemade soap bars and bath products.

First, Learn the Basics of Soapmaking

Before you get started, take a moment to familiarize yourself with the most common methods of soapmaking. Some of these processes are easier than others. Knowing how each one works will help you decide which tutorials you want to tackle.

Make sure to read all the instructions for each soap and take any necessary precautions. Some of these examples use lye, which can burn the skin and eyes if you're not careful.

Create Swirls of Color and Layer Multiple Fragrances

Cold process soap can be made by beginners, but only after learning about how to work with lye safely. Once you get the basics down, coming up with different cold process soap recipes can be really rewarding. This example is eye-catching and smells heavenly

You'll Need:

- Lye
- Water
- Coconut, canola, castor, and sesame oil
- Shea and kokum butter
- Lime, vetiver, and cedarwood essential oil
- Kaolin clay
- Activated charcoal

Cut Up Thin Orange Slices for a Citrusy Soap

This soap recipe is simple because it uses a melt and pour base that is pre-mixed and ready to go. No need to work with messy chemicals! The citrus slices are something you'd only find in handmade soap.

You'll Need:

- Goat's milk melt and pour base
- Silicone soap molds
- Citrus essential oil
- Dried citrus slices

Pair Cocoa Butter and Shea Butter Together

The best homemade soap recipes pair quality ingredients with creativity. Aside from being nourishing for the skin, try to set your soap apart from bars you'd find in the store by adding texture and color.

You'll Need:

- Lard
- Coconut, olive, and castor oil
- Cocoa and shea butter
- Lye
- Water
- Essential oil

- Gold and brown mica
- Exfoliate Your Skin With a Loofah Soap

Loofah soaps are extremely easy to make when you purchase a melt and pour soap base. All you need to do is melt the base and add any extras, cut the loofahs so they fit in the mold, then pour the soap on top of the loofah.

You'll Need:

- Melt and pour base
- Loofah
- Rose essential oil
- Rose mica
- Soap mold

Make Soap Inspired by Your Favorite Tea

When making soap from scratch, try to find a simple soap recipe that utilizes oils you might already have in your kitchen. You can also examine your pantry for other ingredients that would work well in a bar of soap. In this case, green tea is used alongside eucalyptus and lemongrass essential oil.

You'll Need:

- Palm oil and palm kernel oil
- Coconut, olive, castor, soybean, and sunflower

oil

- Cocoa butter
- Lye
- Green tea
- Steeped green tea leaves
- Eucalyptus and lemongrass essential oil

Relax With a Lavender Essential Oil Blend

We love this soap recipe because it is perfect for a relaxing spa day. If you find yourself stressed out and tense, consider adding lavender essential oil to your soap blend for instant relief.

You'll Need:

- Palm oil
- Coconut, olive, castor, and sunflower oil
- Cocoa butter
- Lye
- Water
- Lavender buds
- Orange, patchouli, and lavender essential oil

Sprinkle Some Poppy Seeds Into Your Soap Recipe

Some DIY soap recipes call for color additives like mica or food coloring. This blend is much simpler because the color comes from the essential oil mixture instead of a dye.

You'll Need:

- Coconut, canola, and castor oil
- Tallow
- Litsea cubeba and orange essential oil
- Poppy seeds

Upgrade Melt and Pour Soap With Cinnamon and Cocoa

Easy homemade soap doesn't have to be boring. This particular soap recipe saves time by using premixed soap bases but does require some patience in order to create even layers.

You'll Need:

- Silicone mold
- White and honey melt and pour base
- Cinnamon cocoa fragrance oil
- Vanilla color stabilizer
- Brown oxide color block
- Cocoa powder
- Isopropyl alcohol

Roll Up a Handful of Fizzy Bath Bombs

Not all homemade soap needs to be in bar form. Consider tackling a handful of fizzy bath bombs instead. Aside from the bath bomb molds, you might find all the ingredients inside your kitchen pantry.

You'll Need:

- Baking soda
- Citric acid
- Cornstarch
- Food coloring
- Essential oil
- Water
- Bath bomb molds

Shape Your Soap Into Crystals

This recipe for homemade soap utilizes a glycerin base in order to easily mold and shape the final product. Once a basic soap base is formed, the soap is then cut and carved into small crystals that are used to create a larger crystal specimen.

You'll Need:

- Clear melt and pour base
- Colored mica
- Cosmetic glitter
- Soap mold

- Essential oils

Wash Your Hands With a Soap Gummy

Homemade soap can make simple tasks like washing your hands easier and more fun for kids. If your child is using way too much liquid soap after using the bathroom, consider transforming that liquid soap into a gummy instead.

You'll Need:

- Unflavored gelatin
- Salt
- Water
- Li☐uid soap
- Soap coloring
- Cosmetic glitter
- Soap mold

Use a Bee Mold for Milk and Honey Soap

This soap recipe is so simple that it only requires four main ingredients. Milk and honey is a classic soap combination that is great for the skin, but the soap is infinitely more charming when you use a honeycomb mold like this one.

You'll Need:

- Goat's milk melt and pour base
- Silicone honeycomb mold
- Raw honey
- Yellow and red soap colorant

Learn How to Make Basic Bath Salts

Bath salts make a great gift because they are easy to make and customize. Experiment with different essential oil blends and soap colorings. However, keep the color consistent with the scent. For instance, you wouldn't want to color your salts a mint green if the fragrance is lavender.

You'll Need:

- Epsom salt
- Sea salt
- Baking soda
- Lavender and orange essential oil
- Soap coloring
- Mason jars

Add an Unexpected Ingredient Like Walnuts

Many soap making recipes use common ingredients like milk, honey, and essential oils. However, many food products will work so long as the soap is used within a reasonable amount of time. Got some spare walnuts? Throw them into the mix!

You'll Need:

- Canola, coconut, olive, safflower, and sunflower oil
- Lye
- Milk
- Honey
- Walnuts

Keep the Soap Recipe Simple

It's tempting to want to add a ton of ingredients to your soap recipe, but sometimes simple is the way to go. If you're giving soap as a gift, consider keeping the fragrance something most people would enjoy.

You'll Need:

- Shea butter melt and pour base
- Yellow soap coloring

Lemon essential oil

- Soap mold

Cube Off Some Simple Sugar Scrubs

Sugar scrubs are a luxurious exfoliant that can help revitalize your skin. While you can buy these in the store, they are extremely simple to make. It's possible you'll have most of the ingredients already on hand.

You'll Need:

- Coconut oil
- Shredded soap
- Shea butter
- Lime soap coloring
- Lime essential oil
- Sugar

Add Clay to Your Soap for Acne Prone Skin

An important benefit to making your own soap is that you can tailor the recipe to your skin's needs. If your skin is dry, try a moisturizing milk base. On the other hand, if your skin is acne-prone, consider adding clay to help remove impurities.

You'll Need:

- Melt and pour base
- Bentonite clay
- Soap mold

Combine Oatmeal, Milk, and Honey to Soothe Sensitive Skin

Oatmeal is used to soothe sensitive skin and is a great

addition to any soap recipe. If you find that the oatmeal falls a little flat, the ingredient pairs really well with an almond scent.

You'll Need:

- Goat's milk melt and pour base
- Oats
- Honey
- Almonds
- Vitamin E
- Sweet almond fragrance"

Relieve Sore Muscles With Epsom Salt

One of the most effective ingredients for helping with sore muscles is Epsom salt, and it's easily added to melt and pour soap bases.

You'll Need:

- Epsom salt
- Melt and pour base
- Soap colorant
- Essential oil
- Spray alcohol
- Soap mold

Use Aloe Vera for a Face-Friendly Bar of Soap

This cold process soap has been designed to be gentle enough to use on your face. If you have extra sensitive skin, substitute the coconut oil for babassu oil instead.

You'll Need:

- Water
- Lye
- Aloe gel
- Olive, coconut, sunflower, and castor oil
- Tallow

Use Liquid Bubble Bath to Make Bath Bars

These pretty little soap bars make the perfect addition to any bathtime routine. They work so well in adding bubbles to the tub because the main ingredient is a liquid bubble bath.

You'll Need:

- Baking soda
- Cornstarch
- Arrowroot powder
- Cream of tartar
- Li uid bubble bath
- Coconut oil
- Glycerin

Best Soap Recipes Anyone Can Make At Home

DISCLAIMER

Disclaimer All the material contained in this book is provided for educational and informational purposes only. No responsibility can be taken for any results or outcomes resulting from the use

of this material. While every attempt has been made to provide information that is both accurate and effective, the author does not assume any responsibility for the accuracy or use/misuse of this information.